BEDSIDE
MANNERS

BEDSIDE MANNERS

Your Guide to Better Sex

Theresa Larsen Crenshaw, M.D.

McGRAW-HILL BOOK COMPANY
New York / San Francisco / St. Louis
Mexico / Toronto

1 2 3 4 5 6 7 8 9 D O C D O C 8 7 6 5 4 3

LIBRARY OF CONGRESS CATALOGING IN PUBLICATION DATA

ISBN 0-07-013581-9

Crenshaw, Theresa Larsen.
Bedside manners.
1. Sex.   I. Title.
HQ21.C6913 1983   613.9'6   82-17167
ISBN 0-07-013581-9

Book design by Roberta Rezk

For Ulrika, Brant, and Roger

CONTENTS

14 New Advances in Sex Therapy (and Future Promises) 251

15 Self-Evaluation Questionnaires / Who has the problem, what would you call it, and what can be done about it? 267

Index 295

ACKNOWLEDGMENTS

To Dr. William H. Masters and Virginia E. Johnson for the opportunity to study under their outstanding professional leadership.

To Spencer Johnson, M.D., for helping guide me through the precarious world of publishing, and to Julian Bach, my agent, whose judgment and encouragment were invaluable.

To Audrey and Theodore Geisel, Dr. Morton Shaevitz and Marjorie Shaevitz, Gordon and Ann Getty, for friendship, support, and advice.

For their painstaking review of the manuscript, I thank Purvis Martin, M.D., Katherine Carson, M.D., Steven Kotner, M.D., Bernie Zilbergeld, Ph.D., and Harold Lief, M.D., and especially Lawrence Gross who carefully reviewed and contributed to each draft.

To Ed Hutshing and Igor Lobanov for their willing and timely assistance; and to William Stull for his perspective.

To Mary Erickson and the staff at the Crenshaw Clinic: Jo Kessler, Sallie Hildebrandt, Carlos Miranda, Pat Matterson, Karen Knight, and Sue Steinhoff for loyalty, talent, performance under pressure, and understanding response to deadlines.

To Bob Morey whose meticulous research and merciless critique were exceeded only by the generosity with which he devoted time to this project, to Jeremy Kapstein for his helpfulness, and to Jerry Lilley for his friendship, patience, encouragement, and support during its preparation.

And very special thanks to my patients, whose lives, stresses, and successes motivated me to write this book.

INTRODUCTION

Bedside Manners seeks to improve the sexual and emotional relationship between men and women—enabling them to express joy, experience tenderness, and feel passion.

It discusses modes of communication, not as a set of infallible rules, but as guidelines for allowing individuals and couples to work out their problems—including those outside the bedroom—in order to help them clear the way for warm and expressive intimacy.

It takes into account an individual's relationship with himself or herself. Sex is affected by depression, fatigue, poor self-esteem, anger, and many other emotions. We are not robots. A sexual problem cannot be successfully reversed if one of these problems is responsible and remains untreated.

It deals with the inherent differences between men and women which are matters of physiology, psychology, and cultural conditioning.

Bedside manners—the etiquette of sex—as we know it today often interferes with the natural expression of sex. This book identifies the cultural rituals that are destructive to good sex, and suggests positive alternatives. But these bedside manners are not limited to the bedroom. Sexual manners begin with the kindness and consideration two people demonstrate toward each other in general. They include not only intimacy and emotional rapport, but sexual protocol as well. Sexual manners require that you learn each other's language and develop ways of communicating on a frequency understandable to both of you.

Not all sexual dysfunction stems from psychological problems. Some are the result of physiological conditions—genuine medical problems. As a society we don't know how to judge our own sexual health. We cannot tell a sexual cold from "sexual pneumonia," and we have become a nation of sexual hypochondriacs. At the other extreme, many people have serious sexual problems and do not realize it, or are afraid to admit it. And often the cause of the confusion is a combination of lack of information and misinformation.

For that reason this book gives detailed information in non-technical language on the physiology of sex—his and hers—aimed at dispelling myths and putting people more at ease with their bodies and how they function.

Knowledge is power. It can help you separate those problems that need professional treatment from those you can resolve yourself with the help of an understanding partner. And in some cases, knowledge can remove a "problem" that was really created only by myths and misinformation.

But suppose the problem is one of bodily dysfunction? There's help for those problems, too, in many cases. And medical knowledge of how to cope with such situations is steadily growing. Some of those techniques are discussed in this book and should not be overlooked by those who fear they have no hope of sexual happiness.

This book begins with a discussion of expectations, feelings, communication, and the influence of mood and lifestyle on sex, with practical suggestions to help counteract adverse influences. It then focuses on the specifics of sex—orgasms, erections, impotence, premature ejaculation, ejaculatory incompetence, and disorders of desire—providing the most current information available. It defines what they are, identifies what affects them, and gives specific suggestions on techniques, behavior, and attitudes to resolve problems that occur in these areas.

The next focus is medical. The most recent information is presented regarding the diagnosis and treatment of medical problems adversely influencing sexual function. After a discussion of future directions, the book closes with a series of self-assessment questionnaires which assists the reader in systematically using the material in the book to ask a series of logical questions—Do I have dysfunction? Is it physical or psychological? What can I do about it? This book enables you to explore highly sensitive issues in the privacy of your own mind.

Bedside Manners is intended to help people with good sex make it better. Those who are incubating sexual difficulties will be able to diagnose them early and take steps to correct them. Those who already have obvious sexual problems will receive specific suggestions based on the latest information and research findings.

This book helps you use your natural resources to improve the quality of intimacy in your life. It develops comfort, improves understanding, and teaches men and women to communicate with one another more effectively.

I waited many years for someone else to write this book. I needed one like it to recommend to people in general and to my patients in particular. Some books on sexual function and dysfunction concentrate on psychology, giving generous interpretations and little practical advice. Others focus on medical and biological aspects of sex but are so technical and difficult to understand that the reader becomes discouraged. Other sex books emphasize communications and the relationship without addressing specific sexual issues. And many sex books concentrate on one sex to the exclusion of the other, seeming to neglect the significance of the interaction with another person. Most books give you one feature or the other, but don't address them all. I wanted a comprehensive book on the subject—one that included all the significant factors affecting sexual performance and responsiveness, with the most up-to-date accurate medical information, self-help suggestions, and high doses of basic common sense. Not finding a book that met all these criteria, I was motivated to write this one.

A special feature of this book is the interweaving of the medical, physical, and emotional factors affecting sexual performance. Your feelings, your relationship, your personality, your physiology, and your health all influence your sexual experiences. By the time you have finished *Bedside Manners,* you will be better able to understand and respond to the intricate relationship between mind and body, man and woman, sex and emotions.

In certain areas, I have been purposely provocative in order to challenge our biases and stimulate thought. There are always questions that cannot be answered, or whose answers today will be different tomorrow as our definitions, values, and scientific data change.

In my private practice, I have used humor therapeutically. Men and women have serious problems but need not take every issue seriously in order to solve it. Sex has typically been treated as dreadfully academic or as a dirty joke. Humor, as we apply it to other aspects of daily living, needs to extend to sex too. Although this book deals with very serious issues, I have written it in a way that I hope will make it comfortable and enjoyable—because, after all, that is how sex itself should be.

CHAPTER 1

Great Expectations

The seeds of discontent

The Marriage-Go-Round

Have you ever wondered why people fall in love and then end up having so many problems? Almost everyone you meet today is either premarriage or predivorce, whether they know it or not. How many of your friends who are "happily married" turn up divorced? How many people have you heard announce, "I'll never get married again"? How many of them are still single?

Most people who get married want to be happy. They are not *trying* to make themselves miserable, although it sometimes appears that way.

Things don't always turn out the way they were planned. Our judgment isn't always the best. Our needs are strong and work in mysterious ways. We are the unsuspecting victims of our own personal villains. But that can change.

Why Good Relationships Go Bad

What happens to these promising relationships? Everything starts out well. You like each other. You are interested in his ideas, and he listens attentively to yours. You spend as much time together as you can and enjoy what you do—holding hands, gazing at the moon, movies, picnics, or just doing noth-

---

TABLE I
UNREALISTIC EXPECTATIONS THAT
LEAD TO SERIOUS PROBLEMS

UNREALISTIC EXPECTATION: "Sex should be spontaneous."

SERIOUS PROBLEM: *Infrequent sex and unwed mothers.* If you are waiting for the other person to be spontaneous, you could be waiting a long time. When you don't do any planning, sex usually occurs late at night after the children are in bed, when you are both too tired to have any fun. Next time you are about to have sex, ask yourself: "Do I have the energy to go dancing, play tennis, go to a movie, watch television, read a book?" If you are looking forward to some sleep instead of a good time, you will probably get neither. That is a fertile state for disappointments, hurt feelings, and arguments. Unwanted pregnancies occur when you feel awkward "being prepared."

"I shouldn't have to tell him what I like. He will know what to do." — *Nonorgasmic women, poor-quality sex, and misplaced anger.* When you don't respond to him, you assume he isn't trying, doesn't care, or has no talent. You waste your energy trying to change him instead of doing the very things that could help yourself. When it doesn't occur to you that you are in charge of your own responsiveness, you will look in all the wrong places for help.

"I should be able to make her orgasmic. If she isn't, it must be my fault." — *Impotence and sexual aversion.* He begins working at sex. He tries so hard to please her, he gets cramps. He leaves himself out. The harder he tries, the softer he gets. He eventually starts avoiding sex and/or becomes impotent.

"Don't make an issue over small problems. — *Explosive arguments.* You tolerate and repress irritations. They fester until "the

Wait until they are significant."

"Once you get married, you shouldn't have to masturbate. Your partner will take care of all your sexual needs."

"Love and sex. You can't have one without the other."

"Marriage will make you live happily ever after."

straw that breaks the camel's back." A huge fight begins over something trivial, and everyone later says: "Gee, that was trivial. We shouldn't make such an issue over something so small!"

Affairs. When, as invariably happens, you don't constantly fulfill each other's sexual and emotional needs, you feel deprived. You don't masturbate. You deserve more love and consideration. You wait a long time (for you). If your partner won't give it to you, you'll just find it somewhere else! The lyrics express it: "He won't miss and she won't miss what we're taking here tonight."

Infrequent sex. There are many times when you don't love each other—at the moment. Many women (and some men) will avoid sex if there is an unresolved argument. How many days do you think go by without a disagreement or two? Not many. How do you think that affects your sexual rhythms? This misconception alone can reduce your sexual frequency to twice a month or less.

Depression, relationship crises, divorce. You forget that you were sometimes unhappy before you got married. It doesn't occur to you that you might be just as unhappy if you lived alone, if not more so. Since you were supposed to be happy and you're not, there must be something wrong with the marriage. The relationship becomes the scapegoat for everything that goes wrong in your life—if you drink, if you lose your job, if you get sick. Divorce becomes a way of blaming someone else for all of your problems.

ing. Neither of you has any preconceived notions of what the other person is like. Feelings are communicated. Goals and dreams are shared. Everything appears to be going well at first. Why do so many relationships go downhill from there?

Contrary to popular belief, in the very beginning your relationship is usually as good as it is going to get. The irony is that a couple becomes less and less knowledgeable about one another as time goes by. How can this be, and why does it occur?

Unrealistic expectations and neglect are the prime offenders. "If two people love each other, that's enough. Everything will automatically go well." Unfortunately, it doesn't. You wouldn't neglect a car that way. When you get a new car, on the first day it is the best it's ever going to get. (There are some notable exceptions.) It isn't expected to run beautifully if you don't maintain it and if you never repair it. Maintenance of a car is not all that complicated, nor is maintenance of a relationship. It is hard work, however, to keep things going well, and running smoothly. You can burn up a perfectly good engine by overlooking the oil, water level, or temperature gauge. You can ruin your marriage too, by letting little things slide by.

In a new relationship, there are no resentments, no hostilities, no suspicions. It is totally pure: unspoiled by arguments and problems. Therefore, what there is feels good. All the expectations you have are positive—and you have a truckful of them.

In a seasoned relationship, old hurts and misunderstandings fester. Various mutual hallucinations such as "You don't love me any more, and you never have," "All you care about is sex," and "All you want is my money" have replaced earlier illusions.

Soaring expectations have crashed to earth and changed from the unrealistically positive to the ridiculously negative. A sense of balance? There is none.

The Pleasure Principle

These undesirable changes are no accident. There is no wicked witch's spell. The behavior of couples changes drastically after they get married.

When you date someone, you are doing it because it makes you happy, or you think it will. The person you are dating is doing the same thing—both of you are pleasing yourselves in each other's company. It certainly isn't a case of "Look at that unattractive man. He sure is pathetic. I think I'll make a date with him and help him out, poor soul." Or, "That girl looks lonely. With those horn-rimmed glasses and buck teeth, I'm sure she never gets a date. I'd better invite her out and take care of her because no one else will."

Some people find helplessness appealing. But that is not the general rule. Most people decide to date because there is some kind of attraction—physical, emotional, or financial.

The Sudden Shift

When they decide to get married, suddenly everything changes. These two people stop pleasing themselves and try instead to please each other.

The things they were doing before worked. If this young couple had continued taking care of themselves and each other the way they naturally did while they were dating, the relationship would have continued to grow.

This well-intended "altruistic" shift is often the beginning of the end. Unfortunately, many people are still blinded by the initial rush and unable to see the danger signs.

Do Unto Others as They Would Like to Be
Done Unto

Ironically, the deterioration of the relationship begins by people just living up to what they have been taught to believe: think of the other person first; don't be selfish; the more it hurts, the better the gift. The Golden Rule says, "Do unto others as you would like them to do unto you." If it read, "Do unto others as they would like to be done unto," women wouldn't get fishing poles for Christmas and men wouldn't get purses they don't want to be seen with.

The idea that you will create a successful, lasting marriage by committing your life and energies entirely to pleasing someone you love sounds wonderful—but doesn't work very well, in practice. In fact, it can do serious harm. This and other beliefs we grow up with prevent many relationships from developing their original potential.

The Difference Between Humans and Rats

This brings to mind a major difference between human beings and rats. Rats don't have belief systems. If you put a rat in a maze with four tunnels and place a piece of cheese down tunnel number 4, the rat will explore until he finds the cheese. Then he will go straight down tunnel number 4 until the cheese is changed to another tunnel. The rat will check tunnel number 4 a few more times until convinced there is no more cheese there. Without much ado, he will then go exploring again until he eventually finds the cheese down tunnel number 2. What does the human being do? The human being goes down tunnel number 4 *forever*! Even when there's no cheese. Because he has a belief system. He believes there is cheese there. He must not be doing it right. He goes faster, slower, backward and sideways. He tries harder, but he never gives up.

A man *believes* he can assemble toys, garage door openers, and barbecues without reading the directions. A woman *believes* her husband will divine what she wants for Mother's Day without being told. Twenty years later, she is very angry and still waiting. No cheese!

How Belief Systems Lead You Astray

We all hold many belief systems that we don't even agree with when we take a good look. Many of them are not even on a conscious level. Since these values, belief systems, and expectations help us choose our husbands and wives, they influence our happiness in a very powerful way.

Even though most of us no longer intellectually agree with the following stereotypes, childhood conditioning may prevail at the emotional level. Let's explore a few of them, beginning with what a man wants in a wife and what a woman wants in a husband.

The Perfect Wife

What is a typical man's concept of a wife? What attributes are going to give him the sexual and social satisfaction that he wants from a marriage?

Most men form ideas about what they want in a woman at a young age. They notice how their mother treats their father. They either like it or dislike it. They will want the same thing for themselves, or they will listen to what their father is complaining that he lacks, and want that. It doesn't seem to matter much whether Dad drinks, runs around, or is never home.

A collage of attributes men find desirable includes the following: They would like a woman who is groomed and pretty at all hours, including 3 A.M. She should always be in good spirits and supportive of him, especially when he is wrong. She will be his own special cheerleader whether he is bowling for dollars or running for president. It is a source of pride if she is good at sports, as long as she knows when to lose.

He expects her to anticipate his emotional needs even before he is aware of them himself. He won't have to talk to her much, because she will be able to read his mind. She must understand when he is busy or preoccupied, without complaining, and she should know he loves her without needing to be told more than once.

A good wife is a good nutritionist and a good cook. It is her responsibility to see that he does not end up with a larger abdomen than he had when he was playing ball in high school. She is a good hostess who is nice to everybody he brings home, regardless of his friends' nasty habits (smoking cigars, burning holes in the furniture, telling dirty jokes, etc.). She is also a resident seamstress, a chauffeur, and a bargain-hunter *par excellence* who gets everything at half price. In her spare time, she makes marvelous formal gowns out of bedspreads or old curtains, whatever is handy.

She is not supposed to have a career, unless she has to work to keep the family together while he is out of a job. The man is responsible for supporting the family when everything is going well, but when calamity strikes, she is supposed to come to the rescue and hold the family together until he recovers. She is the

Rock of Gibraltar in a storm. He is the captain of the ship on calm seas. Otherwise, she is welcome to sell real estate on the side or to have some job that doesn't interfere with his needs, wants, wishes, and desires. It must be very clear to all his friends that she is working because she likes to and not because she has to.

She will put him first and the children second, whether the child is vomiting or not. She constantly monitors his needs and, without asking, intuits his every wish. Her needs either coincide with his, or she stifles them.

To complete this list of female attributes is a comparable list of undesirable qualities. A woman resembling any of the following is clearly unmarketable: All men know that good wives don't disagree with them, that they have the final word, and that women who complain are bitchy. She shouldn't ask you to help with chores, especially in front of your friends, be upset if you're late, ask where you have been, like fancy restaurants, order à la carte, or wear expensive clothes. She shouldn't insist on dancing with you (or anybody else) at parties. She shouldn't talk too much except to other women and then, of course, not about you. It's all right for her to have opinions of her own as long as they agree with yours.

Demanding is out. Criticism outrageous. Crying is allowed only if she's hurt herself or you're leaving town. Ideally, then, the male enters a relationship with a woman who is his idea of perfect, and who does not yet show signs of causing him problems later on.

Her Sexual Talents

Sexually, she should respond enthusiastically, preferably in five minutes or less. Saying things like "ouch" or "that hurts" is in bad taste. She should see you as the best lover around, no matter what you do (or don't do). She shouldn't initiate sex when you're not in the mood, but shouldn't leave the burden all up to you either. She is sexually interested and available whenever you are, but never when you aren't. She will want you only, although other men will pursue her mercilessly and envy you your prize. She will moan and groan and call your name (and nobody else's). Most of all, she is to be an angel in the kitchen and a devil in the bedroom—without having had any prior experience, of course.

She must accept that men have frailties. Men have a tendency to let their eyes wander and perhaps have an outside fling or two, but that has nothing to do with their relationship. She must be forgiving and understanding—and faithful.

Armed with these notions, a man scouts for a woman who resembles them. At the same time, he wonders if he shouldn't just forget the whole thing by remaining safe and single indefinitely—a powerful temptation. Meanwhile, he thinks to himself, "I'll keep my eye out and my guard up, just in case."

The Perfect Husband

The woman's job description for a prospective husband is no more realistic. She wants a man who is handsome, strong, virtuous, healthy, clean, wise, gentle, and, of course, a good provider. He should be smarter than she is so she can look up to him. (Taller helps, too.) It is especially exciting if he works hard and is climbing the professional ladder to somewhere, either literally on a construction crew or figuratively in the corporate world.

He needs to be emotionally strong in a crisis, reassure her when she's worried, and be masterful in his problem solving. On the other hand, it's absolutely endearing when he can be emotional and cry, as long as it isn't at the wrong time (like when she's crying too). He can't be weak when she needs his strength and reassurance. He should be thoughtful, considerate, and kind, especially to women, animals, and children. It is perfectly all right if he works hard to get somewhere in the business world as long as he does not neglect her, comes home every night at six, is a good, attentive husband and father, takes out the garbage, helps around the house, and arranges for housekeepers, child care, and travel, while giving her his undivided attention.

She would like him to make all the important decisions, unless she disagrees with him. He is allowed to spend the money he earns on things of which she approves, such as the children, the house, and vacations, but she prefers to have veto power on golf, business trips, and other issues of questionable value. Each year she expects to receive one dozen long-stemmed roses on her anniversary, her birthday, and Valentine's Day, complete with clever poetic cards (better if they are original and written by hand), and various assortments of fine jewelry and furs—without having to ask, of course.

He is there for her whim and entertainment when he comes home from work. He should be prepared to take her dancing or stimulate her with entertaining conversation. Best of all, he should go into extensive details over his problems and concerns so that she can sit, mediate, and advise him on how to handle the major issues in his life.

He shouldn't watch football, play poker, or develop a beer belly. Only bachelors and other undesirables ogle women, get drunk, go out with "the boys." Her husband won't swear, smoke cigars, or wear T-shirts to bed.

His Sexual Talents

He is completely responsible for the quality of their sex life. He will be perpetually erect, even during intercourse. He will be gentle and knowing—a patient, loving teacher. He will know what to do, how to do it, when to do it, how to please her, how to make her responsive, how to attract her, how to make her lust for him passionately. It is not necessary for her to tell him what she likes (that just makes sex clinical and takes the romance out of it). Occasionally she might venture to put a book on sexual techniques under his nose in case he doesn't seem to have gotten the knack yet, but that's only necessary for men who aren't doing adequate research on their own. (Not with other women, of course.)

He must love her faithfully and not stray. If he does, he should have the decency not to tell her about it. And, of all things, he must not get involved with any of her friends. He should constantly lust after her whether she's interested or not and no matter how she looks. She is free to go to bed in hairpins, with cold cream on her face and frownies on her forehead, attempting to sleep on the tip of her nose to avoid crushing her hairdo and the toilet paper wrapped around her head. He is expected to know better than to suggest sex at a time like that.

The Perfect Marriage

We are told very sketchy things about marriage. Save yourself for marriage. Don't get married until you are old enough. Marriage will bring you happiness, if you follow the rules.

If you marry the right person, you will live happily ever after. (No one ever mentions what will happen if you marry the wrong person.) Love will be enough (as long as he has money or a job). She will read your mind and anticipate your every need. He will know how to please you sexually without being told. You will never argue. You will agree on everything, especially on raising children and spending money. In fact, you will think alike, talk alike, look alike, and eventually get a dog with a strong family resemblance.

The Perfect Problem

Are arguments really signs of a bad marriage? Absolutely not! Of course there are arguments, and of course hurtful things are said. Sometimes the first major problem is the very first disagreement. You have been taught that if you love each other, you won't fight. At the first sign of discord, it's home to mother and the marriage is ruined. The disagreement wasn't the problem—the reaction to it was. You start to fear that you made a mistake. The seeds of discontent leading to thoughts of divorce have been planted. Who said "problems bring you closer together"? Having problems is not the sign of a bad marriage. How a couple *deals with* the problems determines whether or not that marriage works.

Be prepared to experience problems. Don't be insulted when they occur. You won't get a vacation from living in the real world by falling in love. Instead of having one set of problems, a relationship has three: his problems, her problems, and their problems—not to mention his reaction to her problems and her reaction to his problems (and her response to his reaction to her problems, and so on).

Marriage is like many things—law school, medicine, housework, teaching, writing, children. If you knew in advance what was really involved, you might never get started. A little bit of ignorance keeps the world turning.

Here Come the Children

About the time you get acquainted with all these expectations, a whole new set of potential problems may arrive to challenge your tenuous grasp on sanity: kids!

Children can affect a marriage in many different ways. Almost everyone is taught that when you have children, it brings you closer together. In fact, children have the power to challenge a good relationship and destroy a bad one. Let us attempt to dispel the illusion that children automatically bring you closer together (except perhaps in self-defense).

Several years ago *Parents Magazine* had a centerfold that was captivating. It was not a Brigitte Bardot or Farrah Fawcett-Majors, but a Supermom with six children in diapers. She was beautifully dressed and immaculately groomed. The kids were teetering on chairs, clinging to vines—six problems in the making. Supermom described her wonderful relationship with her husband and her family. In her spare time, she wrote articles for various magazines as a free-lance journalist. It was more wonderful than believable.

In general, the majority of stresses created by children develop merely from the presence of persistent kids with a lot more energy than you have. Whether you are a mother or a father, it puts your nerves on edge, makes you frazzled, and often irritable. When a couple doesn't compensate by getting more rest or creating more private time, sex doesn't have much chance.

Taking these things into consideration, children present certain challenges. In general, children make bad marriages worse, and good marriages trying. If there is awareness beforehand instead of abject shock after the fact, these issues can be dealt with successfully, and children can be enjoyed.

However, both men and women have such unrealistic expectations of a mate, marriage, children, and sex, that each of them is in for trouble even though neither of them knows it yet.

The Sexual Consequences of Unrealistic Expectations

Instead of responding to their own sexual needs, men and women add to their repertoire of improbable goals. The man is taught that it is his job and obligation to turn the female on, that he will do five minutes on the right breast, five minutes on the left breast, five minutes on the genitals and, by gosh, after fifteen minutes she better be ready because he is. He learns that it takes the female longer to warm up, and that it is his job to make her orgasmic. If she does not respond, it is his failure. That is just like saying he makes her thirsty or sleepy. Listen to the vernacular of sex: "I turned her on. I made her come. I made her." Compare: "I made her hungry. I made her thirsty. I made her sleepy."

The woman learns that the man has a pipeline from God that he is going to bring to bed with him. The man will wave his magic wand, arouse her burning desire, and send her into throes of ecstasy whether she cooperates or not, and certainly without her help. She is supposed to lie there quietly. He must overcome her reluctance, her resistance, her anxiety and awaken her, just like Sleeping Beauty.

These still prevalent attitudes do not generally work. Instead, sex often becomes a chore and a disappointment. Eventually the sexual experience is approached with apprehension rather than anticipation.

Firecrackers, Fingernails, and Other Hazards

Another very common set of expectations come from confusing fiction (the book and movie variety) with fact. Popular novels describe the sexual woman as physically violent, a calisthenic expert and hazardous to your health. As everyone knows, when a woman has an orgasm, if she has the best kind of orgasm, a real orgasm, she gets wound up beyond all control, makes loud noises, convulses, digs in her nails, loses consciousness, and falls off the bed. She explodes inside, firecrackers go off, and music from *Bolero* plays. In a book called *Never Leave Me,* no fewer than three women bit their men on the lips and drew blood because of the frenzied activity of the sexual act.

Sex Can Be Natural and Fun

And with all those unrealistic expectations that we take to bed with us, we expect sex to work! We expect sex to happen naturally. But it simply isn't biologically possible to take over somebody else's natural function. A man can't make a woman orgasmic without her cooperation; a woman can't make a man erect against his will. But that doesn't stop us from going down tunnel number 4. Our upbringing and the belief systems resulting from it prevent two people from using their common sense to satisfy their sexual hunger just as they would to satisfy their appetite for food. Instead of communicating with one another and cooperating with their individual appetites, they are busy trying to do it for each other. It doesn't work that way.

Sex can be natural and fun if you are willing to change the expectations, patterns, and habits that so successfully interfere with it. Throw out your preconceived notions of what a wife ought to be or how a husband ought to act, and discover what you really want. Many disappointments and frustrations will disappear when you develop goals based on your own personal research.

CHAPTER 2

Why Sex Doesn't Just Happen Naturally

Why do two people who don't have sexual problems individually get together and develop one?

Most people agree that sex is a natural function. This statement does not shock anyone. We think of sex as a natural function. We are even willing to talk about it as a natural function, *but we don't live sex as a natural function.* Until we begin to do so, sex won't work naturally. You protest. You are different, you say. I hope so!

There are many examples of how we treat sex differently than all our other natural functions. Let's compare masturbation to eating. People don't quit eating by themselves once they have formed a relationship. Hunger for food often results in eating alone. What about hunger for sex? When people get married, there is an unspoken understanding that it is no longer necessary to masturbate. As a matter of fact, if they are sexually happily married, they shouldn't even want to masturbate. Besides, it's immature. It is a form of juvenile behavior that sometimes persists, but only if you have not adjusted well to sexual life as an adult. If you are not satisfied sexually and it is your partner's fault, that sometimes justifies masturbation, but only as revenge.

*If Masturbation Doesn't Make You Go Blind, Then
Why Are So Many People Wearing Glasses?*

Our attitudes toward masturbation result in inappropriate abstinence or such severe guilt when we do masturbate that we end

15

up feeling bad about ourselves—because of something almost everyone does.

Those who are the most ashamed of masturbating hide in the bathroom, run the water, sing or play music, close the blinds, and turn off the lights. The well-adjusted ones lock the door, make sure everyone is out of the house, hide under the covers, and then do it anyway. A few brave souls wait until he's (she's) asleep and try not to shake the bed. This is quite an art.

One twelve-year-old boy got up in the middle of the night and washed his own sheets. Adolescent boys doing laundry at *any* time should be considered highly suspect.

Another youngster confessed to his mother that his penis was going to fall off because he had been masturbating too much. His penis was a terrible mess—red, swollen, and scraped. She eventually discovered the problem. He had been using her bottle of Pretty Feet (for removing calluses) as a lubricant. It was not really punishment for his sins, but he thought it was.

Can you think of anything most men and women do that almost all of them feel guilty about? It is quite a dilemma. People should either stop masturbating and not feel guilty, or stop feeling guilty and continue masturbating.

Doing It Backwards

If you cut down on food intake long enough, eventually your appetite diminishes. The same is true for sex. Many women, in particular, are aware that the less sex they have, the less interest they have.

And yet, a man still believes he will be more potent if he hasn't ejaculated for a week. It isn't true. He believes he will be able to run faster, box harder, play better football, and feel healthier if he doesn't have sex. For years, athletic coaches enforced the rule of no contact with women the night before the "big game." Too much energy could be lost, they said. Of course, there is no way of knowing how many players masturbated instead. Women think that if they have orgasms with masturbation, they won't have orgasms with intercourse. Nothing could be farther from the truth.

How to Develop a Sexual Problem

Two sexually healthy people get together, and they develop sexual problems. Why does this happen?

The most common reason is the result of a difference in sex drives.

He wants sex three times a week, she wants it once a week. Both are normal but their rhythms and needs are off. Just as individuals have different needs for sleep, sex drive varies, too.

He starts feeling rejected, she starts feeling pressured. Guilt and resentment set in. She withdraws sexually. He withdraws emotionally. Their frequency goes down. They start fighting. That leads to even less sex. After a year or two he's saying, "She's never interested." She's saying, "All he ever wants is sex."

Even if they both wanted sex three times a week, the odds are against both being in the mood at the same moment on the same day. He prefers morning; she likes to sleep in. She prefers evening; he's too tired.

Differences in sex drive are the general rule, not the exception. We also have different preferences in specific sexual activities.

Eating is the only other natural function people do more often together than apart. Our appetite for food varies from person to person. There are individual preferences in the amount and kind of food a person eats. Think of how well different appetites for food are usually dealt with, and compare that to how poorly we often handle different appetites for sex. If your mate isn't sexually hungry when you are, what are the consequences? If you aren't both equally interested at the same time, someone usually ends up with hurt feelings.

No other natural function is expected to occur in synchrony with anybody else's. Mutual orgasm is an exciting goal set by our society and encouraged by Harold Robbins. What about multiple orgasms? And how do you have multiple mutual orgasms?

Doing the Impossible

Visualize a slightly different society. You have two people sitting on adjoining toilet seats because their culture tells them mutual urination is the only way to fly. The conversation goes something like this:

WIFE: "Wait a minute, dear. I'm not ready yet."

HUSBAND: "Can't you hurry up? I've only got a few minutes. I can't wait."

WIFE: "I'm just not in the mood."

HUSBAND: "You're never in the mood. What's the matter with you anyway?"

WIFE: "I'm sorry that it takes me so long. I just don't know what's the matter with me."

HUSBAND: "Well, I can't hold back any longer. You're either going to have to hurry up or wait until next time."

Why We Treat Sex Unnaturally

One reason that sex is treated so unnaturally is that we don't grow up accepting that sex is truly just another bodily function. A natural function is a bodily process that is inborn. It is not artificial, acquired, or assumed. We don't give sex the same respect given to other natural functions like eating, urinating, breathing, defecating, or sleeping. Instead, we treat sex like an illegitimate child. It's there, it's "natural," but it's an embarrassment that we don't legitimize, acknowledge, or accept.

Society does not provide us the privilege of living sex as a natural function. I can't think of any other natural function that is called sin. No other natural function is illegal. California, since 1972, has considered any sexual activity between consenting adults in private legal. In Missouri, it is still illegal to have sex except in the missionary position, and then only if you are married. (Perhaps that is one of the reasons why people say, "I'm *from* Missouri.")

Born Free

Natural functions are congenitally determined at the moment of birth. Sometimes it is necessary to teach a newborn infant how to nurse or to stimulate them to breathe for the first time. However, no one can teach a newborn to suck, breathe, or urinate if that child isn't born with the natural capacity to do so.

Sex is just the same. A newborn infant is born with the capacity to be sexual. Newborn boys have an erection in over 50 percent of the cases before the umbilical cord is even cut. Dr. Masters used to have a contest with himself while he was delivering babies to see if he could cut the cord before the little baby had his first erection. He lost 50 percent of the time. Baby girls lubricate in the newborn nursery within the first two to three hours of life. Both responses are determined biologically. Nobody taught that little boy how to have an erection and nobody taught that little girl how to lubricate. Yet, most parents have seen erections on their baby boys and know for a fact that they occur.

Sex During Sleep

During sleep, the conscious brain has been turned off, but the body works normally, under the control of your involuntary nervous system. Just as digestion, breathing, and heart rate continue effortlessly, so does erection or lubrication.

A three-year-old male child spends 20 percent of sleep time fully erect. At puberty, the erection time increases to 40 percent, where it remains until the boy is about twenty-one, at which time it drops back down to about 20 percent again. By the time a man is eighty, the percentage of time erect has decreased only slightly, to 18 or 19 percent. Assuming a good state of general health, men are erect every eighty to ninety minutes throughout the night, whether they know it or not. Women also lubricate cyclically during sleep. Unfortunately, lubrication and erection are individual responses and not in synchrony with anybody else's. I have known women who lurk awake at night for an opportunity to pounce on the unsuspecting erection. It generally doesn't work because the chances are good he will wake up, and as soon as consciousness returns the erection wilts.

Most men have awakened in the morning with an erection. They assume it is somehow connected with the urge to urinate. He just happened to awaken during one of the ninety-minute erection periods.

The ability to be erect is a birthright. Your sexuality continues to function and maintain itself whether you are asleep or awake. Men have wet dreams during sleep. They are physiological orgasms which are just as real as those occurring in a waking state.

Women also have orgasms in dream sleep. However, since they usually don't have stains on the sheets—as men do—to remind them, they may wonder whether it was "just a dream" or whether their mind is playing tricks on them. Her orgasm during sleep is just as real as a man's. Women often don't recall them—or recall them only vaguely. If a man has a middle-of-the-night ejaculation, there's little doubt about it the next day.

Conscious Control

To some degree, if we so choose, we can prevent, inhibit or delay most natural functions, some for a longer period of time than others. Some people have learned to consciously slow their heart rate or lower their blood pressure, especially if they have been trained in biofeedback techniques or Eastern philosophies.

As we progress down the scale of natural functions, more and more conscious control is feasible. Hunger can be denied for a longer period of time than thirst. Where does sex fall in this spectrum? Somewhere off the scale and into the next room. Sex can be consciously controlled for a lifetime, as demonstrated by the commitment to celibacy of priests and nuns.

One thing natural functions have in common is that if your body stops any one of them, the organism dies. If breathing stops, or urination stops, or the ability to eat and digest food stops, you die. If sex stops, the organism doesn't die, but the species does. Sex is selective, but not elective.

Bedside Manners

All other natural functions get some respect. They are understood for what they are and treated accordingly. We are taught certain manners about other natural functions—when to do them, how to do them, under what circumstances. With sex, we are not taught how to do it. In fact, we are often taught not to do it at all.

Human beings are biologically alike in most major respects. However, depending on what culture you come from or what religion you believe in, the manners you are taught about the various natural functions will be very different.

Every natural function has some rituals associated with it. The more control you have over a natural function, the more manners there are.

Respiration: Can you think of any manners you have been taught about respiration? How about "Cover your mouth when you cough or sneeze. Don't yawn in public. Don't breathe in people's faces. Take breath mints. Don't eat onions unless he does. When in physical competition, don't breathe hard before he/she does."

These manners are so second nature by the time we are adults that one often doesn't recognize that they are cultural and learned.

As natural functions are more easily controlled, there are more rituals and manners associated with them.

Urination: Many rituals govern urination. "Boys stand up, girls sit down. Wash your hands afterwards. Don't splash. Put down the toilet seat when you're done so the girls won't fall in. Close the door." That's America. In many other cultures it's acceptable to urinate against a building or on the street as long as nobody is downwind.

Eating: This natural function is farther down the scale and we have many more rituals associated with eating and many more cultural variations. The utensils as well as the manners differ from culture to culture. "Elbows off the table. Chew with your mouth closed. Don't sing at the table. Keep your fingers out of the butter. Don't wipe your mouth on the tablecloth."

Sex: As we grow into adulthood, we also learn sexual manners of some sort, without even realizing it. "Shower first and wash your privates. It is impolite to squeeze, jump up and wash your hands, or gargle. Don't interrupt in the middle to urinate or answer the telephone (unless you are married), and don't think of anyone else during sex. Ladies first, so please hurry up, but he should try to last as long as he can."

Don't criticize—no hints, no help, no hands—and don't look. Don't talk about sex, except to ask "Was I good?" You must tell whomever you happen to be with: "You are the best (first, only) lover I have ever had." Tell him he has the biggest penis you have ever seen, and that every time is better than the last. Tell her you love her, and be sure to remember her name in the morning.

There are many more sexual manners—some more subtle than others. Unfortunately, the kind of manners most of us learn makes good sex almost impossible.

How to Eat With One Chopstick

In some places, eating with your hands is the custom. In other cultures it's polite to belch after a meal. Not in this one. It is well accepted and well understood that these cultural differences exist. There is usually a tolerant effort made to respect and behave in concert with the rituals of a different culture, if indeed an American finds himself in a foreign country.

However, sex is a totally different matter. Our sexual manners in America are not called manners. They are called values (or religion). They are not only our values but should be everybody else's too. The Eskimos who share their wives are wrong (even if they are warm and friendly). The Arabians who have harems are heathens. The Swedes who live together without marriage are immoral.

A prominent difference, then, between our attitude toward all other natural functions and our attitude toward sex is that cultural differences are tolerated or understood for all the others while sex is marked by intolerance and absolutism.

All of the manners associated with other natural functions may be inconvenient, may be irrelevant, but they don't prevent the expression of the natural function. Whether you're eating with a fork or with chopsticks, the end is met—you get the food into your mouth and satisfy your hunger.

Most manners we Americans have been taught about sex are about as useful as being taught how to eat with one chopstick.

The manners, values, and rituals associated with all of our other natural functions alter them somewhat but don't prevent them altogether. Unfortunately, the things we are taught about sex as children inhibit the natural expression of sex as adults.

We treat sex like the United States used to treat China: it was there, but we pretended it didn't exist.

No wonder we reach maturity with tremendous anxiety over sex. Roadblocks, taboos, frustrations, and guilts are ingrained. It doesn't surprise me that so many people are sexually dysfunctional. I find it amazing that, in spite of our upbringing, so many people manage to have a healthy sex life.

Circuit Breakers: How to Interfere with a Natural Function

We also sometimes interfere with other natural functions. Everyone has a friend or a relative with chronic constipation who is adamant about having one bowel movement a day whether she needs it or not. These people take laxatives and enemas to make them perform the way they feel a normal body should. The end result, as most doctors will tell you, is that they interfere with nature, and create unnecessary medical problems.

Similar problems result from abusing sex, by not treating sex as a natural function. Prostatitis (inflammation of the prostate) is one of the most common complaints that a man will experience if he is not having enough sex, or indeed if he is having too much sex.

The pelvic congestion syndrome is another consequence of not treating sex as a natural function. Women who have irregular or rare sexual tension release may develop congestion and discomfort in the pelvic area. (More about this in Chapter 7.)

A sure way to interfere with *any* natural function is to watch it. If you are eating alone in a restaurant and you suddenly notice out of the corner of your eye that someone is staring intently at you through the plate glass window, things begin to change. You become self-conscious. You can't get all the lettuce in your mouth in one efficient move. Salad dressing dribbles down your chin. You choke on your milk and spill in your lap. As a matter of fact, everybody in the room can hear you chew (you think) and swallowing becomes an unusually difficult maneuver.

As long as you weren't paying attention, and didn't think anyone else was either, you managed to negotiate all of the complex motions involved in eating without a catch. Just being watched really cramps your style.

"I'm not like that," you say. "It doesn't bother me when people watch when I eat." That's good. How about when you urinate?

You probably don't have any trouble urinating at home in the privacy of your own bathroom. However, if I asked you to stand up in front of a hundred people and urinate in a cup while we all watched, do you think you'd be able to do it? You might have a little trouble getting your stream started. Most people would.

Just watching a natural function interferes with it. Sexually, when your partner is saying, "How close are you? Tell me when you're ready to come. Are you aroused yet? Why are you taking so long? Do you think you could hurry a little bit?" Or, "Why don't you slow down. Try not to come so fast this time" and "I wonder why you're not getting hard yet," you will react as you do when any other natural function is being watched. You become self-conscious. Then you begin to watch yourself. It doesn't really matter whether the spectator is someone else or you yourself. The effect is the same.

As a matter of fact, sex between two people can turn into group sex. There is you, and then there is him. There is you watching him, and there is him watching you. Then there is you watching yourself and him watching himself. Suddenly there are six people all concerned about how everyone else is doing. Will goals be met? How are they performing? Who is doing what to whom? Erections and orgasms under these circumstances are very rare.

Pressure is another certain "circuit breaker." Pressure affects all of your natural functions in some way. If you are under great stress or have pressing things to do—deadlines to meet, a party to prepare for with the guests arriving in ten minutes, a job to get to on time in the morning—it will affect your appetite for food, disrupt your bowel habits, or make it difficult for you to sleep.

Sex is no exception. Pressure usually reduces sex drive and inhibits performance. However, if you are anxious, your sex drive may increase. Some individuals under the pressure of studying for an examination will masturbate compulsively and persistently completely out of step with their natural pattern, due to the anxiety. Other individuals become too anxious or too depressed to have sex at all and find that their libido disappears.

What is a normal sex drive?

ANSWER #1: Twice a day to once a month is a normal range for both men and women. Two or three times a week is average.

ANSWER #2: There is no "normal" sex drive. It is normal to have *no* sex drive under many circumstances: if you are tired, depressed, worried, sick, or if any of your other natural functions need attention. It is normal to lose your sex drive if sex has become work, signifies failure, or is surrounded by stress. Much of your sex drive is psychological. If you are enjoying it, you will want it more often. If you are not enjoying it you will avoid it.

The Job of Sex: Why Working at Sex Doesn't Work

"Not me! I never work at sex. It's fun and I enjoy it." But are you sure? The work ethic is so buried in our culture that we don't even notice it sometimes. It even shows in our sexual expressions.

A man worries about whether or not he will be able to "perform," and "works" at lasting longer. A woman tries to "hurry up" so that she won't get left behind. Working at sex doesn't work. Have you ever tried working to get to sleep at night because you have a big day tomorrow? What happens? You lie there wide awake until you finally stop trying so hard, and only then do you fall asleep. When you try to help sex along by working at it, by making it a chore, by trying to time your responses to some one else's norm or by speeding up your reaction pattern to avoid boring or tiring your partner, sex just won't work. It's like trying to hurry up any other natural function. "Hurry up and urinate. We don't have time to wait for you. Everybody's in the car." That kind of pressure inhibits a natural response or causes it to take longer.

Somehow along our evolutionary development our bodies developed in such a way that our breathing, heart rate, digestive system, and sexual machinery all worked naturally (unless some disease process interfered). Sex would work naturally too if bad bedside manners weren't constantly interfering with it.

How Important Is Sex?

A fascinating fact about natural functions is that when nothing is wrong with them, they're not important at all. In our day-to-day, moment-to-moment, conscious living experience they can be taken for granted. They function normally. They function naturally. They don't require our attention. (As a matter of fact, just calling attention to a natural function inhibits it.)

On the other hand, when something goes wrong with a natural function, any natural function, it instantly becomes the most important thing in our lives until it's successfully fixed. If something goes wrong with your breathing (ask any asthmatic), few would criticize you for being preoccupied with the inability to breathe. If you have a bowel obstruction, if your heart is not working properly, if you have a kidney infection, it becomes the most important thing in your life until the problem is solved.

When sex is working naturally, you can take it for granted and pay no special attention to it other than for recreation or procreation. However, when something goes wrong with sex you become preoccupied with the problem, which is normal and healthy—and perfectly appropriate. However, typical responses to your concern are: "You're making too big a deal out of it. Sex isn't the most important thing in life, you know." "I shouldn't care. I should be able to live without it." "It shouldn't be that important. I'm too old anyway." "Why can't I just accept this situation gracefully instead of thinking about it all the time."

You wouldn't say that about any other natural function. You would not chastise yourself for attending to your cold or your chest pain. Don't be so hard on your sex life.

If men and women could actually learn to *live* sex as a natural function, instead of just giving it lip service, most sexual problems would disappear. However, we fool ourselves. We think we are doing so, but it often isn't true.

If you want to test yourself, think of sexual situations that are (or have been) uncomfortable for you. Then compare that vignette to eating or urination. Are you truly living and behaving as though sex is a natural function, or is it just an academic thought to you with no practical application? If you cannot think of any examples, refer to the table of unnatural acts at the end of this chapter.

To live sex as a natural function requires taking a critical look at our "sexual sensitivities," programmed from early childhood. Unhealthy emotional reflexes must be denied, and new patterns put in their place.

To work, sex must not be work. You must let it happen naturally, and cooperate enthusiastically with your feelings without trying to rewrite the script.

A TABLE OF UNNATURAL ACTS

Treating Sex Unnaturally	*Treating Sex Naturally*
	(Food for thought: Define the problem; then take care of it.)
Refusing to have sex alone.	Can you see starving yourself if someone won't eat with you?
	Appetites vary. Respond to them accordingly.
Being hurt if your partner isn't interested in sex when you are.	That is as sensible as being hurt that he or she isn't hungry at the same time you are.
	Find ways to keep one another company.
Being upset if your partner isn't as aroused as you are.	When you are eating together, you won't necessarily eat equal amounts or with the same gusto.
	You each satisfy your different appetites together and enjoy the meal. There is no friction over who eats what. Let sex be that way too.
Trying to have mutual orgasms.	It's like aiming for mutual urination.
	Cooperate with your body. Let yourself respond when *your* feeling develops, not only when someone else's does.

Treating Sex Unnaturally	*Treating Sex Naturally*
Trying to make her orgasmic (him erect).	That is like trying to make someone else sleep.
	You can cooperate and make it easier or interfere and make it harder, but you can't do it for them, or in spite of them.
Losing an erection and worrying that you will never be erect again.	If you had a sleepless night, you wouldn't think that you had forever lost the knack of sleeping. You would assume something was temporarily wrong, and trust that you would be back to normal the next night. If, instead, you worried about not being able to sleep, you wouldn't.
	Sex is like that, too. Trust that the problem is temporary until proven otherwise.
Working hard to respond faster.	Imagine pressuring yourself to breathe faster or urinate more or have bigger bowel movements. You would create one more irrelevant, unnecessary problem in your life.
	Enjoy sex, don't work at it.
Feeling forced to go all the way because you have "led him on."	Would you feel responsible for feeding him if he was hungry? (Possibly you would.) But would you feel compelled to eat for him (or even with him) because your cooking aroused his appetite, if you weren't hungry too? I doubt it.
	Think of your own feelings, not just his. Who led whom on, after all?

CHAPTER 3

Bedside Manners

When Sex Isn't New, Can It Still Be Exciting?

All major disciplines have a key question: In religion it is "Is there life after death?" In sexuality the question is "Is there sex after marriage?"

How can you keep your sex life good when day-to-day living doesn't leave much time for it; children, school, dogs and neighbors interfere with it; your parents still do not believe in it; and every sex book suggests one new impossible position?

The Ultimate Sexual Relationship

The ultimate sexual relationship allows you to participate with your feelings—to express joy, experience tenderness, and feel passion.

However, sexual manners are also important. It doesn't occur to most of us that they even exist. (In some people they don't.) If "you don't know any better," you cannot improve. In fact, if your sexual manners leave something to be desired, it may be obvious to everyone but you.

Bedside manners begin in the kitchen, in the car, at work, over dinner, at a movie, or while you are out with friends. A few cross words at a party can create enough friction to prevent a better kind later that night. How you express your feelings outside the bedroom (and to whom) has a great impact on your sex life, and often determines the quality and frequency.

A Sudden Chill

There are times when sexual intensity wanes or disappears entirely. A specific event may signal an abrupt change.

Sometimes sexual interest drops abruptly. Typical turning points are: immediately after the wedding, after the first year of marriage, during a pregnancy, after the children arrive, the "seven-year itch," aften ten years, and after twenty years.

There are many other landmarks in relationships when sex can turn sour, but the above are the most typical. In each of these situations the precipitating stress is different, but there are many common denominators that contribute to why sex gets bland and sometimes downright undesirable. If the problems are recognized early enough, they can usually be reversed, or corrected.

Red Flags

If you feel that you are missing something sexually, if you feel alone, left out, and are coping with patience, tolerance and "maturity"—don't play the waiting game, these are red flags. Sexual problems may not be recognized for what they are; love is so strong, they seem unimportant; time will take care of them; they shouldn't be allowed to become an issue; she is naive; he trusts he can teach her; he is inexperienced; they just aren't used to each other yet; things will get better; just give it some time . . .

If you have thought or said any of these things to yourself, there is probably a problem brewing. It is not a crisis now, but it will be if you don't pay attention. Here are two important touchstones:

1. If you think there is something wrong with your sex life— even if it crosses your mind as a vague possibility—there probably is.

2. Ask yourself: "If my sexual relationship never changed— if it stayed like this forever—would I be content?"

If your answer to the above question is no, you have some soul-searching to do. What are the problems? You need to know. Don't avoid them, hoping they will disappear. They won't. Face the fact that you are not sexually content. Do something about it now, before it is too late. The longer you delay, the worse it will get. Do not wait until depression and poor self-image set in.

If your answer is yes, ask yourself how your partner would answer the same question. If the answer is also yes, you can be secure for now. Ask yourself these questions again each year. If and when the answer is no, do not be complacent. Solve the problems while they are still small and manageable. Don't drift until a crisis explodes, disrupting everything you hold dear.

Immediately After the Wedding

During the dating and courtship period when a man and woman have sex, it is fun: they both want it, it is slightly forbidden, exciting, interesting, and enjoyable. Most of all there is no sense of duty or obligation.

Those women who are raised to save sex for marriage sometimes run into problems on their wedding night. When that special night occurs, she expects intercourse to transport her to ecstasy beyond her wildest dreams, although she is apprehensive because she has heard that it hurts at first. However, she tells herself that it will only hurt for a little while and then she will have wonderful feelings. Unfortunately, often she does not have wonderful feelings; she is terribly disappointed and wonders if something is wrong with her or if something is wrong with her husband. She lies awake all night in confusion. It must be one of them because this isn't how she was told it would be. She feels defective and inadequate; she also feels terribly alone and afraid to discuss her fears with him because he might think she was criticizing. Intercourse signifies failure to her and she begins to dislike it. As a result she avoids any touching and intimacy that might lead to sex. It wouldn't be fair to lead him on. She loves him and can't lie or fake her feelings. She begins to avoid the whole issue as best she can, for as long as she can.

After the First Year

After the first year the newness of the relationship has worn off. Two people know one another better. They leave the bathroom door open, wander around in tattered clothes, and pass gas aloud. Familiar behavior begins to surface and little irritations erupt. Nylons hang in the bathroom, toothpaste globs harden in the sink, he crunches his ice, she talks too much. Each becomes more critical of the other, and less and less considerate. Attack and defend becomes a pattern that occasionally draws blood. The worst wounds occur because no one is used to being hurt by his or her closest love. Scars form, resentments grow, irritations accumulate. It is also a time when one or the other may experiment with an affair. There is listlessness, boredom, and a quiet blaming of the other person for all of life's miseries. "What happened to the loving, sexy girl I married?" "What happened to that romantic, thoughtful, considerate man I loved?"

During a Pregnancy

Case history: "The first couple of months of her pregnancy were difficult for her. She had a lot of morning sickness and I understood that she didn't feel good enough to have sex. After a few months she seemed to feel better but still avoided me, and I started to suspect her comments were excuses instead of real problems. It just seemed like she didn't want to have anything to do with sex anymore. My father told me that when women are pregnant, they get very emotional and act strangely; but I didn't think that they would lose their entire sex drive. It was a rough nine months, but I figured after the baby came things would return to normal. It didn't change at all. Instead it got worse and worse."

In this case the woman's pregnancy gives her an excuse to avoid sex. Her sex life was not particularly exciting before then, but she was compliant and cooperative, believing that a good wife always accommodated her husband with open arms. The effort was beginning to show when the pregnancy and the symptoms that went along with it gave her a badly needed break from his sexual overtures. When the symptoms of her early pregnancy improved, she felt loath to resume the sexual connection because the absence of pressure had been such a relief. Because she was pregnant, she had a technical excuse to avoid sex without facing the fact that there was something obviously wrong with her relationship. By the time the baby was born, the asexual pattern was established and she continued in her state of relative indifference until her husband could tolerate it no more and brought her to therapy.

Everything Was Fine Until the Baby Arrived

Bill and Ann both described their sex life as wonderful fun until the baby was born. Ann was tired a lot with the midnight feedings and baby care. The doctor said wait six weeks anyway, so Bill was patient. Ann began to notice some resentment on his part when she would wake up at night to look after the baby; and she started becoming hurt and annoyed that he had so little understanding. Comments like "You'll put out for the baby but not me" seemed childish and thoughtless. She couldn't very well let the child starve or mildew in its diapers. Sometimes when they were having sex, the baby would cry and she would get up to take care of it. Bill showed no grace and often turned over angrily and went to sleep; a day of silent disapproval followed. Ann started feeling as if she was being forced to make a choice between Bill and the baby. She was constantly under pressure and tension, and started feeling apologetic for caring for the child. Sometimes she even accused him of being jealous of his own son.

The illusion that children bring you closer together backfires when a young husband and wife find themselves fighting over the very infant that makes them a family.

The first few months of a baby's life are very demanding, especially if there is colic or any of the other common problems to deal with. The first few years can be chaotic while both mother and father are victims of this little tyrant. Mothers bond tightly to the infant; fathers often bond much later, some not until after the child is five or six or seven. Consequently, there can be a great lack of understanding between the mother and father over how each reacts to the child. This discord, in the face of what should have been a harmonious experience, drives the couple apart emotionally and climaxes in the bedroom. Fatigue, irritation, hurt, mistrust, and misunderstanding often replace the sexual liaison. As sex dwindles, so do intimacy and trust. It may take many years to bring the relationship back together. Often a divorce intercedes.

After the Children Arrive

If we were to think clearly about sex and marriage and children, we would notice early clues that suggest children and sex don't mix. The first clue is misleading. Sex and children seem very closely connected, as indeed they are. Children are created from sex and then seem to destroy it.

As the child gets older, there is a greater and greater infringement on private time. Before children arrive, there aren't any major problems in arranging an evening out. There is no need for babysitters and that added expense. There is time to sit and relax over a cocktail after work while reflecting on the day and discussing whatever there is to catch up on. However, when a child is pulling your hair, demanding your attention, running through the room, clicking the television set on and off, smearing greasy fingers on the woodwork, and spilling grape juice on the rug, conversation gets fragmented and peace of mind disappears. How many two-year-olds will sit quietly and listen while Mommy and Daddy talk? Two-year-olds aren't part-time companions—they are there all the time.

The Seven-Year Itch

The restlessness of the seven-year itch is considered a relationship problem, but it is a relationship problem in appearance only. At this time the individual is becoming somewhat discontent with life in general, questioning his or her function and purpose in life, wondering why he or she isn't happier, and so forth. Much of this discontent is aimed at the marriage in general and the spouse in particular. Affairs occur frequently at this stage as this person searches for a meaning to existence and is basically doing research on life's options.

Ten Years

Enter a female-induced relationship crisis. (Refer to Chapter 9.) When the woman is between twenty-five and thirty-five and has been married approximately ten years, she suddenly puts on the brakes, does an about-face, and startles everyone—her husband, her family, and her neighbors, by walking out—with or without her kids. She has everything she could ever want. How could this happen? Her husband is a nice looking young man; he has a good job and is moving up in the world. She has three beautiful children, a nice house with a backyard and a pool, and a maid once a week. However, she also has severe and chronic depression that's been developing over several years. Her toddlers, whom she loves deeply, exhaust her. She feels guilty and unfit as a mother; housework is routine, boring, and demoralizing. Her hard-driving husband (in everything but sex) is rarely home. He appreciates her from a distance; he is usually too tired to pay attention to her conversation and rarely discusses anything of importance with her. He's picky and critical about little things. He appreciates her tremendously, doesn't know what he would do without her, but neglects to mention it. He travels, has business dinners, often drinks a little too much, complains about her spending all the money he works so hard to earn, and alternately feels miserable, abused, overworked, and noble—all at the same time.

She feels guilty and inept, unable to please him, suffocated by the children, hungry for a kind word, crippled by criticism. She has no one to talk to intimately and lives in her private hell. She has tried to get his attention over and over again. He says, "There, there, don't worry about it. Don't be hysterical, don't make such a big issue over every little thing." One day she walks out, disappears, and sues him for divorce. Or runs away with another man with whom she's been having an affair to soothe her wounds.

Twenty Years of Marriage

Enter a male-induced relationship crisis. The man is getting older. He can see over the other side of the hill and is descending steadily with acceleration into his midlife crisis. Glimmers of awareness develop. He begins to realize that he has sold his emotions for logic and reason. Where are they now? He has been on automatic pilot toward goals and achievements programmed in him from early youth. If he has achieved those goals, he's unhappy; and that unhappiness is tragic. If he has not achieved those goals, he's unhappy and assumes it's because he has not achieved those goals. He can see that in his lifetime he won't make the mark he had intended and sees no alternative to failure. His children are grown up enough to provide adult problems: drugs, crime, failure in school. His wife has changed: she is distant and removed—seems to have a life of her own in a world different from his. His success has not impressed her, his failure has not moved her. He is aging and afraid. He has been faithful up to now but decides to have a desperate affair. He leaves his wife and runs away with a younger woman, in search of his past, dreaming of a different future.

How to Revive Your Sex Life

In all of these situations the precipitating stress is different, but there are many common denominators that contribute to why sex gets bland and sometimes downright undesirable. It doesn't have to be that way.

Whether you are just back from your honeymoon, or you have been watching each other turn gray for years, there are steps you can take to keep your sex life exciting. I have heard strenuous objections to the concept that sex can remain exciting or become enjoyable again after many years of marriage. The popular conclusion is that sex will automatically become dull and romance will fade. Some people are dedicated to the conviction that nothing can be done about it, especially those who have decided to solve their sex problems by having affairs on the side.

Sex will become uninteresting if you stop doing all the fun things you used to do before you were married. However, even if you have been in a sexual limbo for many years, your love life can be revived if you give it some thought and follow some practical suggestions. These remedies aren't very complicated;

most of you know what to do—you are just not doing it. Inertia has taken over.

So, get ready to shift gears, and see what happens.

Make time for what matters to you: Reevaluate your goals and make sure that you are acting in accord with your priorities. Most people aren't.

If you are making a lot of money by working very hard but have no time to enjoy it, your efforts are self-defeating.

Get a grip on yourself and manage your time better. If you are chronically overextended with social engagements and work, you are not controlling your environment, your environment is controlling you.

Spend prime time alone together: When was the last time you were alone together for a few hours or an evening, just the two of you? I mean without the children, without company? How many days, weeks, years has it been? Even our lifestyle at home prohibits much personal privacy. The children's room is frequently right next door to the master bedroom and there is often an open-door policy to the bedroom.

These circumstances can be changed. Under usual circumstances, it is terribly important to recognize that the bedroom door needs a lock, that parents need a place of solace while the electronic babysitter does the watching, and an opportunity to be sexual together while training their children to understand they do need quiet time together. If we were to spend half the energy that we spend on toilet training teaching children to allow us, as parents, some private time, our marriages, our sex lives, and our families would be a great deal healthier.

If you train your children to recognize your need for privacy, they will grow up with some idea of how important sexual intimacy is. A few practical hints:

• Put a sign on your doorknob that says DO NOT DISTURB on one side and WELCOME on the other.

• Carve out some prime time, then create some private time with it. A couple should spend at least one evening a week and one weekend a month alone together.

● Take a hotel room in the town where you live and have an occasional mini-vacation without children.

● Get a babysitter to take the children off somewhere occasionally so you can have a quiet evening at home alone in your own house.

In order to provide prime time, you must be ruthless with yourself. There are enough things to do, enough commitments to be made to keep you busy twenty-four hours a day. If you can't say no to some of them, your relationship may be in danger. It dissolves before your eyes as you commit your time and energy to other things, giving lip service—but little more—to how much you love your wife or husband.

Don't hide sex or sneak around: A woman I know was having a terrible time finding the right time for sex. When her children were in nursery school, the housekeeper was cleaning the house—and what would the mailman think if she answered the door in a bathrobe in the middle of the day? He would know what they were doing. She would be so embarrassed.

Creating privacy is one thing. Trying to hide the fact that you and your husband occasionally retire to the bedroom to have sex is not good for the children, not necessary, and generally impossible to do except at a tremendous sacrifice to your enjoyment and sexual frequency.

Children hide sex from their parents. Parents hide sex from their children. Who is fooling whom?

How many of your parents have ever excused themselves from your company to go have sex? Did they ever give the impression that sex between them was something that was perfectly normal, natural, and a parental prerogative?

As parents continue to blackmarket sex and hide it from their offspring, children who become parents relegate sex to something done early in the morning, during "Bugs Bunny" or "Looney Tunes," or late at night once the children are tucked in bed.

Schedule prime time for sex: A couple waits until they go to bed to think of sex. That is usually when they are exhausted, but it seems convenient. After all, you are both in bed and within range. Your clothes are probably off. It is almost effortless—if you could only find enough energy to get started. If you don't schedule prime time for sex, you can't expect the quality you used to have.

If you are exhausted, you will not be in condition to enjoy anything. Physical feelings usually take priority over emotional needs. If you don't even have the stamina to watch TV, don't expect to be very enthusiastic about sex.

Change your routine: Sex gets routinized: it occurs Sunday mornings after church or Tuesday and Thursday nights, in the dark and under the covers. Eating in the dark is not too much fun either. Sexual appetite becomes irrelevant and The Schedule governs frequency.

Even exciting sexual patterns are pretty tiresome, if used every night. Many couples have several sexual rituals or sequences that they enjoy over and over again. The anticipation and knowledge of what to expect next enhances the experience rather than detracts from it. Still, you can vary the protocol occasionally.

Take small excerpts from your sexual routine: a little sex before dinner; hugging and kissing in the shower; champagne, candlelight, and a bubble bath for two; a little lovemaking during commercials, a sexy movie on your home recorder. Tease each other—it's all right. Every interlude doesn't have to be a seven-course meal.

Take the initiative: Why do you suppose two people sit at home, like vegetables, doing nothing they particularly enjoy? They may not be doing anything they especially dislike either, but each person is reluctant to "impose" his or her wishes on the other. Inertia sets in and multiplies itself over the days and the years.

Remember what it was like when you were single? If you had time on your hands, you were busy trying to find something to do with it. You would read a book, or go out, or call up a friend. You would *do* something! You would not just vegetate and stagnate.

To get around inertia, try fantasizing what you would do of an evening if you were by yourself. Start with, "What would I be doing tonight?" Try to become aware of what you really want to do while you can still make changes. Far better to wake up five years into a marriage, decide you're not happy with it, and take steps to improve the relationship, than to put thirty unhappy years into it.

Get back to thinking what you would do if it were all up to you! Once you have something in mind, suggest it to your partner. The most direct way to do this is to say, "I really do feel like going to a show tonight, and there's one I've been looking forward to. Would you care to join me?"

Set the mood: The most neglected aspect of sex, once wedding bands are exchanged, is the backdrop; the stimulating physical setting is the first thing to go. It becomes the bedroom, at night, when you are both tired. There is nothing more subversive to freedom and uninhibited enjoyment of sex than a cold draft, a wandering child, or mood music by Monday Night Football.

Movies and plays are designed to build a mood—laughter, fear, anxiety, buoyancy of spirit, excitement, what have you. Why can't the setting for your lovemaking be equally effective.

Use your five senses. Appeal to them. When you listen to music, notice which songs arouse you and play them before or during sex. Get tape tracks of rainy nights, ocean surf, a crackling fire. If you want to look more beautiful, put soft pink light bulbs in the bedside lamps and install a rheostat. For your sense of smell, experiment from squeaky clean, to very ripe. Use perfumes and aftershave—but not all at the same time. Explore your natural body odors too. For touch, add lotions or oils now and then. Keep one or two candles—little ones, not the tall church-altar or dinner-table variety—on the dresser in your bedroom, or wherever you are. Select the temperature settings, lighting, and background noise, instead of just accepting whatever is available.

Improve your appearance: The next insult to a good sex life is lack of attention to your personal appearance. At bedtime you are getting ready for tomorrow instead of tonight. Women who wouldn't be seen without makeup before marriage put grease on their faces, and put their hair in things that make them less appealing than porcupines. Men who dressed impeccably for dates haven't shaved all day or showered since racquetball, and come to bed in torn boxer shorts, smelling like an old gym sock.

If your bedtime appearance resembles any of the descriptions above, change it. A woman who sets her hair and looks armed for battle rather than for sex might want to change her hairstyle into something she can blow dry in the morning.

A man might want to shave his beard at night and come to bed looking the way he'd like to feel.

Try changing your appearance to fit your mood. It will translate into a sense of well-being and improve your self-image. Apply a touch of fantasy to reality.

Women: Give yourself a temporary permanent by setting your hair in tight little curlers and wearing it that way for a day. "It doesn't look like me," you say. That's good. Perhaps it shouldn't. If you usually wear ruffles and bows, try dressing in something slinky.

Men: If you're a double-breasted suit type, shift to a casual outfit—levis and sweatshirt—for a change. Shake up your self-image a bit. Unleash your sense of humor and act a different part for an evening. It will have a curious effect on your bedside manner, making you more at ease and less inhibited there.

Be practical: Contrary to popular belief, arranging a glamorous candlelit dinner in a romantic setting is not the best prelude to a sexual adventure. Those sensuous liquor ads neglect to mention that after a long, languorous multicourse meal, where the rich foods are washed down with too much wine, good intentions usually turn to sleep.

Ask yourself if you are usually in the mood to run around the block after such a meal. No? Then sex won't be high on the list either.

But don't give up long, romantic evenings. Just have sex before or during dinner. Then, when you fall asleep after brandy and dessert, it's a natural end to a good evening, rather than a disappointment for someone.

Plan your sexual menu: Anticipating your sexual experiences is important. Fantasize a bit, plan an agenda, mull over in your mind what would be fun, what you're hoping might happen, what you'd like to experience.

Objection! I hear: "If you plan it, that's too contrived. It takes all the romance out of it!"

Is it more romantic to lay there like a limp rag, hoping he'll think of something? You can continue complaining how dull sex is, or do something to make it more interesting. You wouldn't dream of giving a party, then asking the guests to entertain you. And yet, when a woman suggests sex, she really means, "Hey, Let's make love!"

Think ahead. We all know that sex is supposed to be spontaneous, but that doesn't mean your brain has to come to an abrupt standstill until The Moment. As a matter of fact, before you were married when life was so exciting, sex and dating was anything but spontaneous. The day was planned, the date was set, the man was thinking, "I wonder how far I can get? I think I'll take her to Lookout Point. Does she drink? Can I afford one cocktail or two? I wonder whether it would be better to get a flat tire or run out of gas?" The girl is thinking, "Gee, what if he tries to kiss me? Or invites me up to his apartment? I hope he does. What will I do?"

The facts are, you planned! You weren't supposed to admit it, and you certainly wouldn't let each other know, but you planned down to minutest detail. You even rehearsed what you would say to each other, including clever comments to cover awkward moments.

Much of the pleasure of the date was the anticipation, looking forward to it. It could even be considered part of the foreplay. Like the fellow who hopped out of bed indignantly and said, "What do you mean I'm a premature ejaculator; I've been thinking about it all day long!"

Try planning out in detail prior to every sexual encounter what you would like as if it were all up to you. Create a sexual menu. Make an effort. You probably spend more time planning your dinner menu for a week than you give thinking about your sexual menu and it probably shows.

Lend yourself: If you are not in the mood when he or she suggests some sex, let yourself flow with the situation just as you would if you were invited to dinner. You may just keep each other company, or your mood might change. Don't assume that just because you're not in the mood to begin with, you won't get in the mood. Be receptive and you'll discover that more often than not your feelings do change. Some of the best and most erotic sexual experiences occur when we are least prepared for them.

Expand beyond your genitals: Sex gets limited to genital experiences. Sensuality is missing as the man and woman zero in on the pelvis expecting mystery and magic. Sex is a total body experience, a total mind experience, or at least it can be. Don't leave out your ears, your nose, or your toes. The areas other than breasts and genitals are worth including for many reasons. Not only can they feel physically good, but the leisure of exploring the body creates greater intimacy and tenderness.

Improve your emotional appearance: Your behavior becomes pretty casual: when you want something you yell, scream, or nag. If you're upset, you cry, gloom, and complain. You wouldn't treat anyone else that way—even your worst enemy. We are more polite to strangers than to the ones we love. You may need to let your hair down once in a while—and there is no better place to do it than at home—but when you behave inconsiderately and are constantly unattractive, it doesn't do much for your sex appeal.

Attention to your emotional appearance is the most important bedside manner of all.

Don't kill him/her with kindness: Although you are perfectly capable of behaving offensively when you're angry, when you are not, you won't tell the other person things that bother you because you think it may hurt their feelings.

A male patient listed among his complaints the fact that his wife had stopped kissing him twenty years ago. While taking the sexual history from his wife, she revealed that her husband had bad breath and was unpleasant to kiss. She had never told him because she didn't want to hurt his feelings. So she solved the problem by not kissing him for twenty years.

It obviously hurt him more for her to avoid his kisses. Sometimes a little hurt in time can prevent a bigger hurt. The easy way out can turn out to be very hard. After a normal dental and medical checkup, the problem was solved with breath mints.

Since he wasn't as aware of his breath as she was, she carried mints and slipped him one when necessary.

Be nice to each other: Arguments are a serious blow to sexual contentment. Since love gets paired with sex in an inseparable fashion, human beings, especially women, are not inclined to participate in sex if there is emotional discord. There are few perfect days, although some are better than others. If a cross word or a little neglect is enough to squelch your sexual interest, sex will become a rare event.

Some couples think that this situation doesn't fit them at all. They don't argue, but they also don't have sex. What is the explanation? Anger and hostility fester, especially in quiet, peaceful relationships. If one person is passive and the other one quite aggressive, there may be a great deal of surface harmony as the passive partner has learned not to antagonize the aggressive one.

Don't Gunnysack: Men and women who gunnysack (store up) their injuries rather than reacting at the time eventually become sexually antagonistic to their partners—whether they realize it consciously or not.

Example #1: The man is domineering, quick to anger, and critical of everyone, especially his wife. She is quiet and retiring. The whole neighborhood wonders how she has managed to tolerate him for all these years. On the outside she seems to, but on the inside she hasn't. The resentment she harbors has neutralized her sexual feelings toward him.

Example #2: She's pushy and demanding. It seems that she is always complaining about one thing or another. She talks and nags and harps while he retreats behind his newspaper and his television set and Wednesday afternoon golf. He never talks back to her or changes the expression on his face. "Yes, dear," seems to be his entire vocabulary. The neighborhood wonders how this nice, gentle fellow manages to bear up under such torture. He doesn't. The accumulation of insults, abuses, and little injuries becomes a barrier. This woman is no longer sexually appealing to him and he avoids any physical contact.

All of these factors lead to an absence of emotional intimacy. It is hard to be soft. Vulnerability between two people is replaced by defensiveness, warmth by distance, and tolerance of the status quo develops. It is no wonder that sex gets dull, routine, and occasionally nonexistent.

The Chemistry Can Come Back

Is there chemistry? Of course there is and it may well be gone, temporarily. But, to create a new chemical reaction you can't sit back and expect sex to occur by spontaneous combustion. The chemistry doesn't just disappear. It gets driven off. Moderate effort, planning, and participation—as simple and straightforward as that sounds—can breathe life into most sexual relationships. If what you truly want is a more vigorous, enjoyable, romantic, exciting relationship, put these suggestions into practice even if you feel a little bit ridiculous at first. After all, it isn't easy to put them into practice or you never would have let them slide in the first place. However, it is possible. You used to do it years ago.

A Deeper Look

Feelings and behavior—change one and it affects the other. This chapter has emphasized the value of changing your actions in order to change your reactions. This approach can have great impact. But it doesn't stand alone. Superficial formulas for whipped cream, Saran wrap, and sexual toys often backfire. The emotional aspects of sex cannot be neglected. On the other hand, until you are rested, comfortable, undisturbed, interested and interesting, no matter how much love there is, you may prefer sleep.

When he says, "Were you awake?" and she says, "Was that you?" it is time to brush up on this chapter.

CHAPTER 4

The Sexual Troika

Your mental health, self-esteem, and sex—one won't work without the other. How depression, chronic exhaustion, and poor self-image lead to sexual problems and what you can do about it.

If you have a poor self-image, are often depressed, or have sexual problems, you are about to develop the "sexual troika." That is not a *ménage à trois* or group sex. A troika is a Russian sleigh drawn by three horses. And like those horses, low self-esteem, depression, and sexual problems are harnessed together.

The sexual troika begins in one area, but affects all three. You can't have one for very long without the others!

Like dominoes, if you knock over one, the rest fall down too. Let us look at some examples in each category.

- It begins as a sex problem: His impotence depresses him (and her). He no longer feels like a man.

- It begins as a depression problem: Her depression makes her uninterested in everything, including sex. She would rather sleep anyway.

- It begins as a self-esteem problem: He feels inadequate because he can't hold a job. She is overweight and unhappy with herself. Their poor self-esteem leads to depression. Sexual interest and responsiveness disappear.

The Only One You Are Fooling Is Yourself

Sexual problems erode an otherwise good relationship. It doesn't matter whether the difficulty is infrequent sex, lack of responsiveness, impotence, premature ejaculation, lack of lubrication, the absence of orgasms, or no sex at all. Whatever the problem, it causes trouble in other areas.

No matter how hard a person tries to pretend a problem doesn't exist, it is there. It will grow and fester, eventually destroying the good things between two people—until nothing is left.

Few sexual problems disappear by themselves. The more you neglect them, the worse they become.

Even if you can't admit to yourself that you have a sexual problem, it depresses you, makes you defensive, and destroys your self-image. Eventually, you may be forced to face the issue, but by that time you may have lost the person that you love.

The Sexual Consequences of Depression

The sexual consequences of depression aren't noticed at first. Sex is the most vulnerable of all natural functions. If an individual is depressed, the first appetite to go is sex. But the change often goes unnoticed. Frequency of sex usually diminishes. Not being in the mood is explained away by other things: being too tired, working too hard. It is rarely recognized as a symptom of depression in time to prevent the sexual troika.

Depression first leads to loss of interest in sex. If it persists, responsiveness will also be affected, producing impotence or the inability to experience orgasm. By that time, you need a sex therapist, a psychiatrist, and your own personal cheerleader. There is a lot of work to be done.

Masked Depression

Depressions range from mild to severe, with some individuals who are thoroughly aware of their misery, and others who insist they are not depressed.

If you think you're not depressed, you may not be. Or, you

may be experiencing a masked depression. Ask yourself the following questions:

- Am I sleeping well at night?
- Am I generally irritable?
- Do I wake up in the morning without enthusiasm for the day?
- Am I tired most of the time?
- Am I drinking too much?
- Is the Valium running out?
- Have the highs disappeared from my life along with the lows?
- How often do I really feel good instead of just okay?

Depression and a sense of helplessness go hand in hand. When a woman feels as though no matter how hard she tries, or what she does, she can't keep up with her chores or solve her problems, she becomes depressed. When a man feels trapped by a job, unable to make his wife happy, and struggling to earn enough money to provide for his family, he feels helpless to change or improve the situation. Naturally, depression results.

Impotent men are usually depressed, and depressed men are often impotent. Impotent men say that their sexual problem preys on their mind through almost every waking moment. It clouds their whole life.

Emotional Exhaustion

Depression is a state of emotional exhaustion, similar to physical exhaustion. If we could treat depression the way we treat physical exhaustion, there would be far less damage.

If you push yourself too far physically, your body starts to feel terrible. After running one too many miles, for example, you're not sure that you can take another step. If you knew you were going to feel that bad for the rest of your life, you would want to die. However, you realize that rest, relaxation, and a good night's sleep will make you feel good again in the morning—and ready to run a little farther the next time.

We often overextend ourselves emotionally without recognizing it. Life is full of pressures and stresses which are quite capable of driving any normal person into overload. When that certain threshold is passed, one feels so bad, so depressed, so miserable, that life may seem not worth living.

Unfortunately, most people don't recognize those feelings as symptoms of emotional exhaustion. Consequently, they don't realize that with a little rest and pampering they'll feel fine again. Instead, they assume there's something seriously wrong with them and become even more depressed. They may drive themselves to do more and more, in the hope that just getting a little more done will make them feel better. Instead they become more depressed.

Depression Is Depressing

Are you getting depressed because you are depressed? People feel inadequate for being depressed and become more depressed. Consequently, depression often becomes self-perpetuating.

When everything is going well, we're busy wondering, "When is this happiness going to end?" When everything is going poorly, we're convinced that it's going to last forever. A very double-standard point of view. If you are just sad for today, that's bad enough. But as soon as you say, "I'm going to feel this way forever," you have magnified your problems.

If, instead of criticizing your feelings, you could say, "Well, I am clearly overextended emotionally. I need to rest and take better care of myself so that I can feel good again tomorrow," the depression wouldn't last so long.

Depression is also contagious. Most people don't think of it that way, however. If you are living with someone who is gloomy, sad, negative, unhappy, and critical, it is hard to remain cheerful yourself. This is especially true if you are in love with a depressed person: you become depressed being around him (or her), but also become depressed just thinking about the other's unhappiness.

The Terrible Whys

What is the first thing most people ask themselves when they recognize that they are depressed? Why! Why am I depressed?

The "why" is important, but it isn't necessarily useful in dealing with depression. If you don't know why, going through a random list of negative things can only be upsetting.

However, let's say that you know why you're feeling upset. Does knowing why you are depressed change it? Sometimes, but often it does not.

If there is a "good" reason to be depressed, knowing why is not going to be useful. If you are newly widowed, recently divorced, or fired during a recession, the reason is obvious, but knowing why doesn't make you feel any better. It is normal to be depressed under those circumstances. Indeed, it would be abnormal not to be.

Antidotes to Depression

While depression often requires professional treatment, the following self-help techniques are often effective.

Instead of asking *why*, there are two questions that can help: "*What* am I feeling?" and "*What* can I do about it?" No judging, no self-condemnation. Just a practical let's-fix-the-problem-whatever-it-is approach.

The answer to "What do I feel?" is "I feel sad and depressed." The answer to "What can I do about it?" is more challenging.

Change the stage: In order to help yourself change your mood, you first need to change the setting. Even actors who must cry need to think of something sad to make it happen. At the moment, you probably feel like sitting in a dark room brooding by yourself. But if you wish to feel happier, you must put yourself in a setting that allows you to feel better.

You can't change your feelings directly. You can't say, "I refuse to be depressed. I will be happy," or, "I will be miserable." Have you ever noticed that when someone close to you has had a tragedy, it is difficult for you to be empathetically miserable if you have just had a very happy event occur in your life? Your best friend broke a leg and you just won a million dollars. It's impolite to be happy, but you just can't help it. You can't easily will a feeling away.

In order to bring yourself out of a sad mood, place yourself in an environment where you usually feel happy. When you do this, chances of your becoming happier are strongly improved.

So ask yourself, "When I feel good, what do I usually like to do?" It may be to go to a movie, visit with a friend, read a book, watch TV, go jogging, take a walk in the sunshine, play tennis or . . .

Improve the present: Even God can't change the past. Since you can do little to change the past, and the future hasn't happened yet, set your mind to working on improving the present. That way, your future will be an improvement on the past you would like to change, rather than a continuation of old patterns.

Concentrate on changing the present but don't disregard what you have learned from the past or discard your hopes and plans for the future. Trust that if you take good care of the present, your future will take good care of itself.

The choices you make in the here-and-now will influence your future relationships and experiences. Knowing how you feel is critical—but not enough. You must exercise good judgment. And remember that while you are not responsible for having a feeling, you are responsible for the actions you take. You alone, and those you care for, will experience the consequences.

Exercise: One of the best natural antidepressants around is exercise. Although your instinct may be to isolate yourself from others, the best remedy is to force yourself to go out and do something. Anything, even sex, just so it makes you physically active.

Your resource list: The best time to think of things to do is when you're feeling good. Pick a day when you are not depressed to write down a resource list of things that you enjoy doing. Try to think of twenty or thirty items, then put the list aside for easy reference the next time you are feeling sad.

Three gratifications a day: Rate your overall state of mind on a continuum from cheerfulness to misery for a week. Make a list of all the things you do each day. Then, rate those activities from a minus ten (utter misery) to plus ten (bountiful euphoria). If most of your activities are in the minus zone, it's no surprise that you are depressed—you are not doing anything you enjoy. Next, make a list of your greatest pleasures—things that bring you pure joy, that have no redeeming value or ulterior motive. Pure gratification could include playing a spirited game of tennis, sunbathing on a soft beach, a warm bubble bath, a cup of tea, reading the Sunday paper, having a massage, or watching a football game. If tennis is something you do for exercise and really don't enjoy, it shouldn't be on your list of gratifications.

Expand your list of twenty or thirty items, including both five-minute pleasures and some that take all day. Keep your list handy and do two or three of them each day. Refer to it when you're feeling sad or depressed and *force yourself* to do at least one. You will find yourself reluctant to get started, but will be amazed at how the depression will lift once you do.

Refer again to the list of things you do daily and rework your schedule and your activities until you get almost everything in the plus range. It isn't easy but it can be done—and is well worth it.

On the other hand, if you won't be nice to yourself, insist on mistreating yourself, and refuse to take good care of yourself, it's not realistic to expect others to treat you well either.

Escape to: One of the most strenuous objections to the gratifications list that I have heard is that making what the objectors call a cheer-me-up list is not healthy because that means you are escaping the real problem, rather than facing it. Nonsense!

There is a world of difference between escaping *from* a problem and escaping *to* a pleasure. Sleep is a good example. When people become depressed, some sleep. They sleep to escape their problems. They get more tired than usual and sleep longer. That type of sleep is not restful.

On the other hand, if you are depressed and unhappy, getting extra rest could be a positive and productive choice—not to escape, but to treat your emotional exhaustion properly. In fact, next to physical exercise, sleep is our best natural antidepressant. Sleeping for a few hours to treat your state of mind, if it is escaping to a brief rest instead of escaping from the problem, will be healing rather than harmful. As a matter of fact, if you don't get adequate rest, as depressed people often do not, you will continue to be depressed no matter what you do.

The fine line between escaping to and escaping from lies in the attitude behind your behavior.

Who Is Secure?

Everybody has some degree of low self-esteem, but some people mask their insecurities better than others. We are raised hearing, "Don't do this, don't do that. Sit up straight. Study harder." How can anyone growing out of childhood through adolescence and into adulthood, possibly feel adequate, much less secure? No one feels 100 percent good, all the time.

The Gruesome Twosome: Body Image and Sexual Adjustment

If a woman doesn't like the way she looks, no matter how gorgeous she appears to someone else, she will have difficulty developing physical intimacy.

A man, who thinks he is too short, too thin, too bald, doesn't have enough muscles, or isn't athletically talented, will not feel secure undressed in the presence of the woman of his dreams. A perceived defect, no matter how small, can have big consequences.

Some people solve body image problems by turning off the lights and pinning themselves under the covers, but that limits sex to nighttime, unless you are willing to move to Alaska.

Penis and Breast Envy

There has been much talk about women having penis envy and men having breast envy. However, that is not what I mean here. A man may envy another man's penis because it is bigger, longer, harder, or more talented—but mostly because he thinks it is more desirable to women. Women envy other women's breasts because they're bigger, firmer, rounder, more pointed, don't need a bra, and bounce (or don't bounce, if you jog). Many women are convinced that all men want women with big breasts. Men are firmly convinced that all women want men with big penises. No matter how one's partner really feels, the message is unlikely to get across because the mind is stuck.

If you think your penis is too small or that your breasts are too small, how sexually secure can you be? Your sexual self-image will affect your ability to be relaxed with a partner, and will lead to inhibitions that create problems in responding.

Americans have great difficulty accepting compliments. We go to great lengths to hold onto our conviction that something is physically or aesthetically wrong with us. I call this the "Marilyn Monroe syndrome"—referring to the attractive woman who doesn't think that she is beautiful. People tell her how lovely she looks, but she has a special talent for distorting any positive comments. "Don't you look beautiful today." (She's just saying that to be nice.) "I love your hair fixed like that." (She's obviously being catty.) "You look marvelous in that outfit." (Boy, does she have bad taste.)

Tell a man he looks handsome and what happens? Does he say, "Thank you. I'm glad you think so." No. He pretends he didn't hear it, or acts like you have insulted him.

Anyone can, with stubborn effort, cling to negative images of themselves. Marilyn Monroe was an outstanding example. Even the world's admiration is not enough if you do not have self-confidence.

How to Keep Your Self-Esteem Low

1. Insist on feeling bad about yourself no matter what other people say. Turn their comments around and take them in a negative way. It will work every time!

2. Blame yourself when things go wrong, but don't take credit for your accomplishments. If things go well, attribute it to luck.

3. Criticize yourself frequently and hope that someone will disagree with you. (They usually won't because they assume you know best.)

4. Let your physical appearance go, and then look in the mirror frequently and be disappointed.

5. Seek approval from others, then disagree with them.

6. Be harsh or aloof so no one will know you are lonely.

If you are good at feeling bad, the results are predictable. You will form relationships with people who make you feel worse.

Remedies and Solutions

There are some simple steps that can be taken to help improve your self-esteem.

Believe what others say to you: Agree to disagree. You have your own opinion of your adequacies, abilities, looks, and worth. Now, give other people the freedom to think differently, to have different tastes, to like things about you that you might not like yourself. If your boyfriend says that you look beautiful in that dress although you don't like it yourself, say, "Thank you. I'm glad you think so." If your wife thinks you're handsome, enjoy the fact that she thinks so, even if you don't.

Set your own standards: Stop looking to someone else for reinforcement. If you don't have it on the inside, you won't find it—even if it's there—on the outside. Ask yourself who you are living your life for. We often behave as though we are living it for someone else. For example: In a singles bar, both men and women are worried that no one will find them attractive. You would feel more at ease if you realized that you are there to find someone to please you, not to be pleasing to others. Don't settle for less just so that it won't look as though you have been rejected. If someone turns you down, assume that they have bad taste!

Be your own therapist: Take good care of yourself, but most of all listen to all of the advice you give to other people and begin taking some of it yourself. Become the center of your own universe again. If you treat yourself with some respect, other people will start doing so.

Start acting as though you feel good about yourself now: Don't wait until you feel good about yourself to change how you behave. You will discover that changing your behavior in fact changes your attitude. It may seem artificial at first, but after a short time it will become natural.

Pay attention to your appearance: Get a new haircut. Buy some attractive clothes. Go on a diet. Join a health club.

Develop a talent: Find something that you're good at and do it. It will give you self-confidence.

Feel positive: When a glass is filled to the midline, the pessimist will call it half empty, the optimist says it is half full. Both are correct, but the consequences are different. The "half empties" don't feel good about themselves or anything else. The "half fulls" have a head start on filling the rest of the glass.

Recognize your achievements: Tell yourself you are making progress. Compliment yourself on your successes. Treat yourself the way you would a young child whom you're trying to encourage toward greater achievement: lots of approval, lots of compliments, no criticism. Censor any unhealthy talk. Don't allow private conversations with yourself such as: "I did a lousy job on that. I'm never going to get anywhere. I look terrible. I'm too fat. I'm getting old and ugly. I have no will power and no self-discipline. My life is miserable. I hate myself." Don't allow yourself to indulge in verbal self-flagellation. That type of talk is guaranteed to depress.

Warm fuzzies and crooked strokes: A crooked stroke is a compliment with a zinger, such as: "That was really smart—for a blond." A warm fuzzy is a pure, unadulterated compliment, such as "I love you," or "You are beautiful." Avoid crooked strokes. Warm fuzzies are money in the relationship's bank. Make a few deposits each day. Capturing in words the positive things that you feel reinforces their presence in your life, and helps fend off the negatives.

Start taking risks: You have nothing to lose! With a poor self-image, you feel like you can't do anything right—so you don't. Get rid of that idea and start acting as though you are capable of doing things. Take a few risks, small ones at first: initiate sex, go somewhere alone, join a group, start a conversation. You will discover that most of them work out. Face whatever things you think you can't do and take a step in that direction.

Controlling the Troika

It doesn't matter which of the three categories—sex, depression, or low self-esteem—initiated your problem. The best way to solve it is to work on all three areas at the same time. Working in tandem—just like the three horses pulling the troika—the situation can be reversed in a remarkably short time. Trying to work only on one area in hopes that the other two will go away seems logical, but doesn't usually work. If you tackle all three simultaneously, you can take charge of the troika and change directions.

CHAPTER 5

Feelings

The missing link between man and woman—he says it is a sexual problem, she says it is an emotional problem. Who is right?

The Chicken or the Egg?

He says it's a sexual problem. She says it's a relationship problem. If he would only be nice and considerate, she would have sex with him more often. He would be much nicer to her, he says, if she had sex with him once in a while. It's a Mexican standoff. Both dig in their heels. You first! It has become a matter of principle. There is no question about who's right (except in the other person's mind).

She feels that if he really loved her he would be acting differently. He feels the same way about her.

They are both right. It is both a relationship problem and a sexual problem. But, the man won't go to a marriage counselor, and the woman won't go to a sex therapist. A stalemate occurs before they can even get started.

The best approach is to work on the problems in the sexual relationship and the emotional relationship simultaneously. If a problem in one area lasts long enough, it eventually leads to problems in the other—and you end up with both.

Different but Equal

It is recognized that both men and women can have personality traits usually attributed to the opposite sex. Nonetheless, men and women often think, feel, and behave differently. Many factors have come together to exaggerate these differences. They are raised separately together—from the toys they are given to play with to the accomplishments they are encouraged to pursue. There are also hormonal differences—testosterone that makes men aggressive and estrogen withdrawal that makes some women depressed during their periods. Biological differences are evident in strength, size, and shape.

Recent studies on the development of the right and left hemispheres of the brain have found anatomical differences between the brains of men and women. These remarkable findings suggest a biological explanation for some of the differences between the sexes, such as the male aptitude for math and the female aptitude for languages. One of these biological differences is illustrated by patients recovering from a stroke that has affected their speech centers. Women can sometimes talk again by training the other side of their relatively undifferentiated brain. Men, whose right and left hemispheres are more specialized, have greater difficulty doing so.

Learn From Each Other

Men and women could both benefit from becoming a little more alike, with no worry that they'll ever become the same. They could help each other to do so in very meaningful ways. Men could learn to become more familiar and conversant with their feelings by letting a woman be their guide. For example, ask a woman's advice on how to handle an emotionally charged issue instead of giving into the reflex of burying it or ignoring it.

Women could learn to cope with life better by doing the opposite: notice the techniques men use to prevent themselves from fluctuating emotionally. Ask a man how he succeeds in putting upsetting issues aside, without becoming overwhelmed. Discover how good it feels to take action and become a better problem solver.

Men's and women's feelings are alike, and are understandable to one another probably 80 percent of the time. We all know fear, happiness, joy, sadness, enthusiasm, grief. The manner in which we express these feelings may be different, but the feelings are shared.

Then there are times when men and women have no subjective frame of reference for each other. For example, a man doesn't have a vagina or a clitoris; a woman doesn't have a penis. A man will not ever subjectively experience a female orgasm. She will never know what it feels like to have a penis or an erection. Because these are physical differences, the point is not debatable. Emotional responses, like physical feelings, can also be markedly different in certain instances. It isn't essential to know whether the cause is cultural, chemical, or biological. It is necessary to respect these differences and learn to cope with them.

Because of these subjective reactions, it is necessary to express the full scope of your feelings in order to understand one another. You can benefit from each other's help as you follow the guidelines in this chapter.

Hidden Feelings

Feelings! Everyone has them, yet our real feelings are often the most carefully guarded secrets—even, sometimes, from ourselves.

Emotional feelings for the man and sexual feelings for the woman are usually masked by layers of training and social conditioning. Men are often at a loss when asked to reveal their emotional feelings. Women are similarly uncomfortable, embarrassed, or unaware of their sexual feelings.

Men: They don't express their emotional feelings with ease. Society has given them permission to show only happiness or anger. Other feelings are there but rarely expressed. As a result of not discussing feelings, men often don't recognize in themselves the full scope of what they really do feel. Since decisions often get made without taking their feelings into full consideration, the choices are frequently the wrong ones. Once a decision is made however, a man doesn't like to change his mind—which puts him in a terrible fix if he was wrong in the first place.

From early boyhood men make more strenuous efforts to control their emotions than do girls. The inappropriate erection embarrasses them. One of their emotions often shows in their pants. To stop the response, they must stop the feeling—hiding it even from themselves. They also learn to disregard many of their other feelings. Women have no such obvious indicator.

So, when he won't tell you what he is feeling, it isn't because he doesn't have any emotions. It isn't because he is insensitive. It isn't because he's closing you out. It isn't because he doesn't care for you. It is usually that he is so far removed from his feelings that he doesn't realize himself what is stirring underneath until much, much later (if ever)—when it is sometimes too late.

Since men often can't readily verbalize their feelings, they express them in other ways. Most men express intimacy, love, and caring quite easily through touching and sex. That is their familiar medium of communication. They are as versatile physically as women are verbally. During or after an argument, a man will reach out to hold you and soon find himself feeling sexual. This is his way of saying, "I love you. I care. This argument isn't as important as it seems." The woman misses his point entirely and rejects him harshly, saying, "You animal, all you ever think about is sex. Have you no sensitivity?" He does. You're just not noticing.

Women: They don't express their sexual feelings easily. They have been conditioned since birth to be ladies. All of the sexual feelings that a woman might have had are channeled into the more "acceptable" category of romantic feelings and love. She is taught, beginning at a very young age, that she is expected not only to control her own sexual feelings but to control those of the man as well. That requires a great deal of emotional discipline. It is much easier for her if she succeeds in not having sexual feelings at all. And eventually, although her sexual feelings are still there somewhere underneath, she has successfully buried them.

On the other hand, women can express emotional feelings *ad nauseam*. Unfortunately, some women still can't make decisions or take action as easily as a man can. Generally, they wait for the man to make the move, and then criticize whatever he does.

The man loses status points for expressing emotions; the woman loses status points for being sexual. Therefore, most men express intimacy through sex and most women express intimacy through words. Often, the more she cares for a man, the more enthusiastically she will talk to him.

But ask her to describe what she wants sexually and chances are she will be speechless—or tell you something so vague that it is useless. Most of the time she doesn't know. If she does, she's uncomfortable telling you.

Passing in the Night

Men and women often pass each other in the night. They are communicating on very meaningful levels, but neither one can listen well on the other's frequency.

Complicating matters further is the fact that men and women often judge each other's methods of communication. She calls him insensitive and uncaring because he won't talk to her. He calls her hysterical and irrelevant because she talks too much. She accuses him of being interested in her only for her body. He accuses her of wanting him only for emotional security.

Mutual Appreciation: You're in the Same Boat. . . Almost

If, as a man, you feel awkward and embarrassed when you try to verbalize your emotions, you can appreciate how many women feel when they try to express themselves sexually. If, as a woman, you feel uncomfortable in expressing your sexual feelings, you can better understand how many men feel trying to talk to you about all the things you want to hear.

Are You Having Someone Else's Argument?

There are many male/female patterns that clash: shopping, electric blanket settings, and thermostat temperature settings, to name a few. In a store, she wants to look around, he wants to buy something quickly and leave. He wants to sleep at arm's length, she wants to cuddle. He wants the windows open in winter, she has the electric blanket on high in the summer. He is angry with her. She is furious with him.

Chances are you are having someone else's argument. Many issues are repetitions of the same disagreements your parents and grandparents used to have. You may think you invented it, and maybe it was your original idea, but it probably wasn't. Your neighbor, the grocer, and the president have had the same battle. But you suffer just as much as if you owned the copyright yourself. There are many individual exceptions to these rules, but if you happen to be one, I am sure that you know others who fit the pattern.

THE GET TO THE POINT! ARGUMENT.   A very typical male/female conflict is the "get to the point" argument. She thinks out loud. He thinks quietly. She expresses her thoughts. He expresses his conclusions. He's waiting for the punch line. It hasn't occurred to her yet.

The woman says, "How can you have given that so little thought?" He has given it a great deal. The man says, "Get to the point." She's trying.

THE "TALK TO ME" ARGUMENT.   She says, "Talk to me." He says, "Not again!" Her request drives all the words from his mind. He feels ridiculous and can't perform.

Have you ever noticed that men can talk to each other without many words, understand exactly what they're saying and agree wholeheartedly with each other? When a man tries to say the same thing to a woman, it takes him much longer to make her understand, and then she often disagrees with him anyway.

A woman can speak with another woman in half-sentences. A man overhearing the conversation may exclaim, "What on earth are you two talking about? It makes no sense at all." The women try to explain it to him, using paragraphs and paragraphs—and he still doesn't understand. "Women," he'll say. "You just can't hope to understand them. And if you do, you're in serious trouble." They are speaking Greek to him.

THE "LEAVE ME (DON'T LEAVE ME) ALONE WHEN I'M SICK"
ARGUMENT.   A man and woman under stress often have different needs. This leads to numerous problems: the woman will do
for the man what she thinks he wants, judging by her own needs
in that circumstance. That backfires rather badly when their
desires are different. Example: When a man is sick, he usually
wants to be left alone. He appreciates being given some creature
comforts, then left in peace to lick his wounds and heal in
solitude. He does not usually like to have a fuss made over
him.

Naturally, when a man is sick a woman will hover over him,
offer him chicken soup, pester him with conversation and her
presence. Eventually, he gets so frustrated and furious that he
yells at her and drives her out of the room. She runs out crying,
feeling misunderstood and abused. He's lying in bed saying, "I
wish I weren't so sick. I'd rather be at work. Why can't she
leave me alone? My God, that woman is impossible!" They are
rehearsing a very traditional argument.

When the woman is sick, the man knows exactly what to do.
He's going to treat her just the way he would have wanted to be
treated. He will show her how to do it right. He ignores her.
Leaves her entirely alone. Shuts the bedroom door and stays out
of the way. He won't sit by the bedside, hold her hand, or crowd
her at a time when he knows she'd really feel much better being
by herself. He leaves. She's crushed. How could he neglect her
when she needs him so much? He obviously doesn't care for her
at all, or so she thinks. Doing the wrong things for the right
reasons can cause problems.

EMOTIONAL REFLEXES.   Many emotional reflexes of men
and women have been conditioned in separate ways. When men
get angry they are primed for physical combat and often have to
restrain or discipline themselves from participating in a fight.
Women rarely lash out physically, beyond a slap across the face,
no matter how angry they become. A woman may cry "at the
drop of a hat," but many men endure tremendous emotional
turmoil without tears.

New emotional reflexes are difficult to acquire as adults. One
woman studied self-defense and became quite expert at it. She

had a black belt in karate. One night after work, a hand reached out from under her car and grabbed her ankle. She had the skills, but not the automatic fighting reflexes to set her into physical action soon enough to use those skills effectively. She hesitated, was overpowered, and raped.

How Can You Tell If You Are Having Someone Else's Argument?

Real trouble develops when you take sex-linked arguments personally and seriously—as though they were your very own. There are a number of clues that will let you know that the argument is not a "personal" one between you and your partner—rather, that it is someone else's argument, that it is a male/female pattern argument.

If you are repeating your point over and over and still not getting through, you are probably having someone else's argument. If you are not listening to each other but just defending your views and trying to get your partner to agree, it could also be a male/female pattern argument.

A sign that you are in the advanced stages of male/female pattern argument is when the man is trying to undo the woman with logic and she is trying to conquer him with hysteria. It's time to stop. You won't get any farther on that argument. Save your energy and think about the issue again in the morning when you feel calmer.

There is no "solution" to male/female pattern arguments, or they would never have survived these many generations, but there is a "resolution." When you realize you are in such an argument, stop and listen. Stop trying to convince the other person of your point of view. Neither one of you is "right." Agree to disagree. Say "I think this is one of the areas where we have no common ground. I'd like to stop arguing and see if we can negotiate a practical solution, even if we don't agree."

There are times you will simply not understand each other. Bear in mind that it is hard enough to understand yourself. Sometimes you simply won't understand your mate. Let it pass without making it more of a problem than it already is.

What Color Are Your Blues?

Depression is another emotion that men and women tend to react to differently. Women have more typically overt depressions; the kind that are obvious to them and everyone else. Men more typically experience "masked" depressions. They are not consciously aware of being unhappy even though they may be severely depressed. They cope, they function, but they are without joy. Often they do not realize the degree of their despair until they finally feel good again.

The man who abruptly leaves his wife and family and changes jobs, all with little warning to anyone around him, has just recently become aware himself of how miserable he has been. With the conscious knowledge of his unhappiness, he tries to change everything at once—in a vain attempt to make it better.

A depressed man may become chronically angry and irritable, or quietly withdrawn. He may use alcohol to dull his senses, or retreat into his work to avoid his problems.

A depressed woman often becomes emotionally unstable. Her moods show in her actions: She stops taking care of her appearance, gains or loses weight, cries with little provocation, blames others for her problems, becomes chronically fatigued, and can't seem to get anything accomplished.

She tells the man her problems, describing her fears and her inadequacies hoping for reassurance—which she usually doesn't get. He, a problem solver by nature, immediately comes up with a list of suggestions for her on how to solve the problem. If they don't work, his next step is to prove that the trouble doesn't exist. In his repertoire are the following phrases.

1. "You can't mean that a little thing like that got you this upset." (This indicates that from the beginning the problem has been silly and trivial and has no legitimate reason to exist. The problem is solved if he can talk her into the fact that it didn't exist in the first place.)

2. "If you hadn't spent the money in the first place on this useless washing machine, it would never have broken and you wouldn't have this problem." (He is proving that she was stupid, that it is only logical that she should have this problem, and therefore it is unreasonable for her to be depressed.)

3. "There is absolutely no reason for you to be this upset." (If there's no reason, then there can't be any depression, right?)

4. "You are being completely irrational. No one could possibly get this upset just because I was an hour late for dinner." (If his behavior was reasonable, then that automatically means her reaction is irrational if it is about his behavior.)

5. "You are always so emotional. You get upset over every little thing that goes wrong." (Which means that you are obviously defective and if you could only fix your problem these things wouldn't worry you so much.)

Men usually don't show depression in such obvious ways and consequently the woman doesn't have as much opportunity to comment.

All Feelings Are Valuable

Feelings exist whether you like them or not. They are not good or bad. All feelings—whether pleasant or unpleasant—are valuable, even depression. An unpleasant physical feeling such as a headache gives you important information about yourself. It may say: slow down, stop reading, take an aspirin, see a doctor, maybe you need glasses. Emotional feelings also give you information to respond to and go into action about.

Feelings are triggered by current events, but their depth and nature is based on all your previous experience. Just as you are not directly responsible for your feelings, neither is any other person. Who you are, how you feel, and your relationship with that person has more to do with your reaction than what is said. If someone tells you that you are fat and unattractive, your feelings will differ depending on who says it. You may be annoyed by the comment of a stranger, while the same words from your partner might hurt deeply.

Feelings are rarely logical. They are more likely to be capricious and change without warning—sometimes for no apparent reason. You feel very irritable or sad. Suddenly the sun comes out and you, too, feel shiny and bright.

*The Fearsome Foursome: How to Find Your Hidden
Feelings*

In order to make the best decisions you must know how you
feel. That is your data base. Jumping into action without being
aware of everything you feel invites unpleasant repercussions.

Recognizing the scope of feelings you are experiencing is
important. Even more crucial is that some feelings can mask
other feelings. To uncover hidden feelings you must slow down
and ask yourself some questions: What am I feeling? When did
the feelings begin? Are there other feelings present?

Feelings fall into two basic sets of categories. There are recognized and unrecognized emotions, immediate and delayed reactions.

Often, the first emotion we become aware of is not the first
emotion that we have had. Think about the last time you were
angry. Some typical examples that can trigger a good bout of
anger are: your teenager comes home two hours late from a
date; your wife (or husband) overdraws the checking account; a
car cuts in front of you on the highway; your husband accuses
you of keeping a messy house; you stub your toe.

The result is normally anger. However, the anger is usually
the result of other feelings or sensations that aren't even noticed
at the time. In fact, at least one of the following four feelings
may precede anger:

FEAR
FRUSTRATION
EMOTIONAL HURT
PHYSICAL PAIN

One or more (or all) of them are there whenever anger occurs. Look at the examples given above and try to imagine what
you might have been feeling before the anger in each instance.

1. Your teenager comes home two hours late from a date.
   a. *Fear* that the child was hurt or kidnapped.
   b. *Frustrated* by not knowing what to do.
   c. *Hurt* that she (he) would be late, knowing that it would
      worry you.
   d. *Pain* from the headache you developed from worry.

2. Spouse overdraws checking account.
   a. *Fear* that checks have bounced.
   b. *Frustrated* because it has happened many times before.
   c. *Hurt* that he (she) wasn't more careful and considerate.

3. Car cuts out in front of you.
   a. *Fear* that you were almost killed.
   b. *Frustrated* that there are so many dangerous drivers on the road.

4. Husband says you keep a messy house.
   a. *Hurt* that he's not pleased with your work.
   b. *Frustrated* that you can't get it all done.
   c. *Fearful* that you won't be able to satisfy him.

5. You stub your toe.
   a. *Pain.*
   b. *Frustration* with yourself for being so clumsy.

What you thought was just plain anger had several other feelings associated with it.

Look back at the last time you were angry and try to pick out which of the four feelings preceded your reaction. Men usually cite frustration rather than fear or hurt, perhaps because frustration is a less disreputable feeling than fear. If frustration is all you have found, look again and ask yourself specifically: Was I a little bit hurt? Somewhat fearful or apprehensive?

You may have difficulty finding the preceding feelings once you are angry, if the experiences have happened over and over again; for example: Your husband tells you you're overweight or your wife tells you you're insensitive. You have heard it so many times by now, that it simply makes you angry. Twenty years ago, when he or she first made that remark, certainly your feelings were hurt. The way to uncover feelings that you had before anger gripped you is to try to remember what you felt like the first time it happened.

Dealing With Anger

Anger is a powerful emotion. It can be coercive and manipulative.

Anger also is a very uncomfortable emotion to feel. It usually hurts the one who's angry much more than the target—who only gets glancing blows. The person who is angry is uncomfortable full time. So, how do we lessen the anger, especially in a caring relationship? The first step is to realize that you don't have to become angry in order to change someone's behavior. Often, merely expressing the *other* feelings you are having is enough. To the daughter who comes home late you say, "I'm hurt that you didn't call. I'm frustrated at having told you so many times to be home on time. And I was terribly afraid that something had happened to you. You're grounded for a week."

Expressing the fearsome foursome can dissipate anger very effectively, while communicating the exact nature of your feelings.

Anger can be expressed productively or destructively. If you hit your thumb with a hammer, the first feeling is pain. To throw the hammer through a plate glass window, which you will have to repair later, would be a destructive action. A more productive course could be to yell and scream, leap up and down, make a momentary fool of yourself; then walk to the refrigerator, wrap your thumb in ice, and take a couple of aspirin.

It is important not to "repress" anger, nor to express it indiscriminately. The answer lies in expressing the full scope of your feelings to your spouse, partner, child, or friend. This tactic can often bypass the anger altogether—while neither expressing nor repressing it. It simply resolves the issue.

Try it the next time you find yourself becoming angry. As soon as you recognize any signs of anger—irritation, annoyance, resentment, withdrawal—search for the preceding feelings. Express them instead, and notice how it will often dissipate your anger.

Anger and Sex

There is a direct relationship between anger and sexual difficulties. Anger is subversive to sex. It is quietly destructive. It can gradually ruin the best sexual relationship.

A man who expresses anger loudly and explosively intimidates the woman in his life. She doesn't feel treasured, valued, and loved. Her tenderness and softness changes to hurt withdrawal. She may remain socially pleasant for fear of precipitating a temper outburst, but she usually stops communicating sexually and often loses her ability to respond altogether.

The man who doesn't become outwardly angry tolerates a great number of minor annoyances. He is the "peace at any price" man. His wife can nag at him, criticize him, harp at him, and it doesn't seem to ruffle his feathers. On the inside, however, he festers. He doesn't really like the way he is being treated, but doesn't feel the "little things" are worth making into major issues. From day to day, he absorbs these minor insults, doing nothing about them. It is a great surprise to him when he cannot get an erection during sex. It is really not surprising at all. The stored resentments and frustrations he experiences as a result of the way his woman treats him makes her emotionally and sexually quite undesirable to him. Unexpressed anger very effectively neutralizes this man's libido.

It is clear that anger and resentment, whether expressed or unexpressed, lead to sexual problems, particularly if it is an ongoing or long-standing problem. Burying the anger buries your sex drive right along with it. Lashing out in anger buries your partner's sex drive just as effectively. Therefore, there must be another alternative—one that allows anger to be dealt with appropriately without destroying your own sexual interest or your partner's. Expressing your hidden feelings is the key.

On Making Decisions

Your actions will be determined by the decisions you make. There are important factors that must be taken into consideration in order to make sound decisions. These are:

1. Your feelings
2. The feelings of those you love
3. Your own physical and emotional well-being
4. Your short-term and long-term best interests
5. Your extended self

In becoming aware of your own feelings, it is important not to disregard everyone else's.

Beware of Personal Growth

The take-care-of-yourself-no-matter-who-you-hurt philosophy has, hopefully, run its course. Personal growth at any price has cost many a lot: their families, their sanity, and sometimes their fortune. Still, there must be an approach somewhere in between martyrdom and selfishness, and there is. It is based on common sense—a resource that often gets forgotten in our hurry for instant solutions.

You're Not to Blame for Giving Yourself Cancer

Some extremist philosophies suggest that in one way or another, we bring upon ourselves every disaster that occurs. If you crash your car, you must have wanted to kill yourself. If your child is a behavior problem, blame the thoughts you had during your pregnancy. And then there is the ponderous question: What did you do to give yourself cancer?

Self-blame is a misguided attempt to get and establish control over one's life. The reasoning goes like this: if anything that goes wrong is our fault, then, of course, we should be able to prevent problems, fix everything and make it right. Wrong!

Back to common sense. If you don't take care of yourself physically and mentally, you'll be in no condition to take care of those you love. If you insist on martyring yourself for your spouse and children, you will be so miserable that they won't want to be near you. If you insist on driving yourself hard professionally to support your family, you won't see them much, may become an alcoholic, and will probably end up with a heart attack before your time.

A mother who is taking care of a sick child must ensure that she herself doesn't get sick, or someone else will have to take care of both of them.

You cannot count on any one else to take care of your physical and mental health. That is your responsibility alone. However, some of your decisions may distress those you care about. I am not suggesting you be "selfish." Selfishness implies that you do what you want with no consideration for anyone else's feelings.

Self-responsibility merely means to act in your own best interest, having carefully considered the effects of your actions on others. You recognize that choices you make are your own. You must weigh the short-term and long-term consequences of your actions. You cannot hold others responsible for the consequences. But it is counterproductive to *condemn* yourself when things go wrong, even though you accept the responsibility for having made the decisions. (No one has a crystal ball. You can only make the decision you feel is best at the time: you will certainly experience your share of mistakes.)

Under ordinary circumstances, no one can do anything to you without your cooperation. For example, if you have been married to an alcoholic for twenty years who has "made you" miserable and unhappy all that time, one must ask, "Why did you stay?" You answer, "I had no job, five kids to feed, and I was afraid he'd beat me. Besides, he might have killed himself if I left."

So you chose to stay. For some reason it was psychologically or physically easier for you to stay than to leave. The decision was yours. Perhaps you had no easy choice to make, but choice it was. No one did it to you without your help. Many people, under the illusion that someone else is controlling their lives, don't exercise the control that they could. They miss many opportunities to improve their circumstances. Nonetheless, that doesn't mean that they are to blame for every mishap that occurs. It simply means that we don't necessarily function at our peak effectiveness—especially if we attribute to someone else more power over us than he or she actually has.

To be effective you must recognize your active and your passive choices. Active choices are ones that you make for yourself; passive choices are ones you allow or force someone else to make for you (i.e., a man unhappy in his marriage, but without the courage to face the problems, has affairs, leaves evidence for his wife, who then leaves him). In general, active choices tend to be better for you—although, of course, there are exceptions.

Weigh your short-term and long-term best interests and make a decision accordingly. Your short-term best interest will sometimes be the opposite of your long-term best interest: eating a hot fudge sundae when you're trying to stay on a diet, or staying up late at a party when you have to work the next morning. The decision then depends on the price you are willing to pay. In most cases, however, your short-term and your long-term best interests are compatible.

Your Extended Self

In addition to considering your own short-term and long-term best interest, you need to consider the effects of your action on the ones you care for. Imagine two concentric circles. The smaller one is your nuclear self: the physical and emotional *you*. The surrounding circle includes everyone you care for. Call this one your "circle of love."

The people you care for are not determined by *their* need to be loved. Everyone in the world is lovable to someone, or so I hear, but you love a select few. They are defined by your personality, your value system, your nature. Consequently, the people you love and care for are an extension of yourself. They are the product of your needs, wants, cares, loves, and desires—and become your extended self.

If, through your actions, you hurt someone you love, you indirectly hurt yourself. It is therefore not in your own best interest to hurt, upset, or harm someone you love.

If, however, your physical or emotional survival is at stake, you must make the best decision you can under the circumstances, weighing the degree of your need against the distress you might cause those you care for.

For example: If you are in poor physical condition and decide to start an exercise program to improve your health, it may deprive someone of your time and attention. In this instance you might decide to continue exercising in spite of your partner's objections; it is in both your best interests in the long run.

Informed Consent

Making a decision that affects others can complicate your life if you don't discuss it with them beforehand. Some decisions are excellent, but their execution can backfire due to the lack of cooperation if your partner is uninformed or surprised. Remember, he/she doesn't necessarily think like you do.

In order to send thoughts, feelings, and messages across the "sex barrier," you must learn a common language, stop reading between the lines, and be very clear.

If you speak in half-sentences, give hints, or express vague, incomplete thoughts, your partner will usually succeed in misinterpreting you. You know exactly what you mean, but don't assume that he or she does. "I'm tired" can mean "Let's have sex," "Don't bother me," "I want some sympathy and appreciation for how hard I work," or "I want to go to bed and sleep."

The next chapter will help eliminate the guesswork.

CHAPTER **6**

"I" Language

Expressing Your Feelings—The Key to an Intimate Relationship

Why does our intelligence and common sense desert us when it comes to sex? First of all, we don't know how to talk about sex. We don't have a vocabulary for sex except tongue twisters like "cunnilingus" (oral sex) and swear words. As a matter of fact, there is a nonvocabulary for sex. As we grow up, we are taught that sex is something *not* to talk about.

Tell It Like It Is!

There is today, however, a great deal more open discussion about sex. It lulls us into believing we are advanced and sophisticated. It gives us the illusion that our children won't have the sexual problems we had. We talk about sexual attitudes in general, sex in the movies, sex in the streets, and the affairs and exploits of neighbors and friends. We *don't* talk specifically about ourselves very often, if at all. Trying to solve a sexual problem by talking about everyone else's problem except our own is about as effective as going to a doctor to get help for indigestion and discussing someone else's eating habits.

77

Monday Morning Quarterbacks

Here is an example of how we talk a great deal about sex, but we don't communicate with our sexual partners in a way that counts. Example: breakfast conversation the morning after the night before:

WIFE: "I really enjoyed myself last night."
HUSBAND: "I did too. Did you come?"
WIFE: "No, but I almost did."
HUSBAND: "Is there anything else I can do to help you out?"
WIFE: "Well, if you'd just done thus and so a little longer. I was almost there. I think it would have happened that time. I was so close."

Next night, the wife is thinking, "Gee, I sure hope he remembers what I told him. Well, he's doing that all right, but right now I'm really feeling in the mood for something else. I wonder how I can get him to stop doing that and start doing this."
Next morning:

HUSBAND: "Did you come last night?"
WIFE: "No, but I would have if you had done this instead of that."
HUSBAND: "But that's not what you told me to do."
WIFE: "Yes, but I didn't want that any more."

Next night, husband does this instead of that. Wife thinks, "Gee, I wish he wouldn't press so hard; it's starting to hurt. I hope he stops pretty soon. I'm getting raw."
Next morning:

WIFE: "That was feeling good for a while, dear, but then it started getting uncomfortable and I wish you had stopped earlier."
HUSBAND (in a rage): "First you tell me to do it longer, then you tell me not to do it so long. Why can't you make up your mind? I don't think it has anything to do with what I do or what I don't do. You're just frigid!" (Storms out of room in anger, stage left.)

She could talk all around the issue and give him a lot of advice on what he should have done last night and what she hopes he will do tomorrow. But she can't tell him *during* sex!

That's when it's happening (or not happening). Since tomorrow often changes and he is more likely to do the right thing at the wrong time, these morning-after discussions don't communicate very useful information. To be effective, communication must occur at the time, so that if her needs change, which they usually will, he is informed immediately. She must develop the ability to tell him what she wants when she wants it, not two days later. Tell it like it is! You can't post-mortem an orgasm. Nothing that you tell him tomorrow will give you an orgasm tonight. Monday morning quarterbacks don't change the score.

I Could Have Told You So

If they had been able to talk to each other about these things, they wouldn't have needed a therapist. This is simple common sense—rational, obvious information on how to solve a communication difficulty. It does not take decades of education, a Ph.D., or an M.D. to figure it out.

The Verbal Void

It is possible to be direct without being harsh. But couples usually settle for being very unclear with one another. They fear that information and discussion will make sex clinical and take fun out of it.

The vagueness with which people interact gives rise to a great deal of attempted mind reading. You try to read between the lines in order to figure out what the other person really wants. Even if he or she tells you, you won't listen because you think you already know. When mind reading is the major form of communication, sex gets pretty dull. You are going to do just what you are sure the other person wants, whether they want it or not. You won't vary from the theme even if they ask you to. You know better. In the meantime, the other person is being just as rigid with you. Flexibility, spontaneity, and ingenuity are out.

For a man and a woman to share their sometimes different feelings requires clear communication and patience. Understanding and cooperation develop from a willingness to learn about and from each other, and a recognition of the differences.

Having differences is inevitable and, indeed, desirable. Without them you would not be challenged or stimulated. How you cope with these differences determines whether you have serious problems or not.

Making Feelings Work for You

No one can know how you feel unless you tell them. Mind reading is at best unreliable. They may guess, and may even be right most of the time, but they will never know when they are wrong unless you tell them, and they listen. "I" language is a way of talking to one another that leaves very little room for misunderstanding.

Two-year-olds use "I" language very well. "I'm hungry," "I want a cookie," "I love you," "I hate you." You never have to say to yourself, "I wonder what he meant by that?" But when he goes to school, one of the first things he learns is, "Don't say 'I.' Don't start your sentences with 'I.' "

He learns to become tactful (untruthful) and civilized (manipulative). Instead of saying, "I want to go to a movie," he says, "Wouldn't you like to go to a movie, Dad?" or "There's a good movie playing at the Guild Theater." Now he fits in. He is communicating just as vaguely as everybody else. You can't figure out what he really wants from what he is saying, so you read between the lines. Second-guessing and interpretation become second nature after a while. "You" language is well established. Instead of believing what you hear, you believe your own analysis of what is being said.

In order to make feelings work for you, *you must express them to someone else.* Feelings can be expressed in many different ways, some useful, others invariably confusing.

HE: "Where would you like to go for dinner tonight, dear?"
SHE: "I don't know. Where would you like to go?"
HE: "Whatever you want to do is fine with me."
SHE: "I'd like to please you."

Four transactions later, they have accomplished nothing but tossing a hot potato back and forth. (Whoever catches it also gets the blame if things don't work out well.)

(HE thinks: "I know she likes spaghetti") and says, "How about Italian food?"

(SHE thinks: "Chinese food is his favorite") and says, "How about Chinese food?"

(HE thinks: "I had Chinese food for lunch, but if she really wants to go there, I'll take her") and says, "Wonderful, let's go."

(SHE thinks: "I'm not too fond of Chinese food, but since it makes him happy, I'll go) (Exit, stage right.)

They end up going out to eat where neither one of them wants to go—each thinking he or she is pleasing the other one.

Lights up in a somewhat garish chrome-and-vinyl restaurant dining room:

HE: "The service is slow."

SHE: "I only came here because you wanted to. You know I don't like Chinese food."

HE: "What do you mean? It was your idea in the first place."

The argument flourishes. They are both wounded by their own good deeds, energetically accusing the other.

Methods that rely on second-guessing what your partner really wants usually backfire. This frustrates all communication. Why talk if, no matter what you say, your words are not believed.

There is a better way.

Effective communication contains five simple, but necessary ground rules:

1. Say what you mean.
2. Be clear.
3. Believe what you hear.
4. Trust that you're both on the same side.
5. Listen carefully.

Say What You Mean

"What do you want for dinner?"

"I don't care—anything will be just fine."

"How about burnt fish?" (Anything is not just fine.)

"What would you like for Christmas?" he says.

"Surprise me," she says.

"Here's a twelve-gauge shotgun, a fishing pole, and a vacuum
cleaner." (Surprised?)

Simplify your life and be honest in your communication. Say
what you mean and mean what you say.

Be Clear

SHE: "I'm tired." (She means, let's have sex.)
SHE: "I'm tired." (She means don't approach me.)

The same words are used, but the meaning is very different.
Misunderstandings are inevitable under these circumstances.

You know what you want, but won't tell, hoping he or she
will figure it out from vague hints. Even when this method fails
time and again, you don't give up. You get angry instead. If you
don't generally get what you want, chances are that you aren't
being clear about your needs.

Believe What You Hear—Don't "Hear" What You Want to Believe

"Why don't you ever talk to me?"
"Well . . ."
"You don't ever communicate with me or share your feelings. If
you loved me, you'd take more of an interest in what I think
and feel."
"I do love you."
"No you don't."
"Yes I do."
"You hate my mother too."
"No I don't."

This conversation is futile.

He doesn't talk to her because she doesn't believe anything
he says. She has her own interpretation of every thought he has.
She is immune to his words. His reasons and his feelings are
irrelevant.

"What's wrong?"
"Nothing."
"I can tell you're upset by the look on your face."

"I'm really just fine."
"Is it something I've done?"
"I'm not angry, God damn it!"
"Yes, you are. You're raising your voice."

By that time he or she *is* angry. A self-fulfilling prophesy has occurred. Refusing to believe what you are being told creates problems that didn't exist, except in your mind, and makes them real.

Trust That You're on One Another's Side

"You're thirty minutes late!"
"But I had to stop for gas. Then I couldn't find a parking place."
"Why didn't you plan ahead?"
"I didn't think the gas was so low."
"If you had any consideration, you would go to the trouble to think
    of these things in advance."

You must trust that the other person is on your side, and would not hurt you on purpose—just as you would not set out to hurt them. When problems occur, you must be secure that they were accidents or unavoidable. Deal with the consequences instead of attacking each other. Otherwise, you will be the victim of perpetual suspicions and insecurities.

Listen Carefully

"You said you didn't want to take the children on this vacation."
"No I didn't. I said I didn't know if we could afford to bring them
    along."
"I distinctly remember your saying that they were too much trou-
    ble and we should leave them at your mother's."
"I said that if they weren't too much trouble, Mother might be
    willing to take care of them for us."
"No you didn't! You. . . ."

This argument is an argument over who said what to whom. The real issue has gotten lost. There was no one there to help you remember what was said. You did not tape the discussion. No one can prove whose memory is more accurate.

If you wish to conserve energy and stop fighting, there is a way to bypass this detour and stick with the issue.

Avoid saying, "I said," or "You said." Eliminate those terms from your vocabulary and substitute, "I meant." You cannot remember precisely what you said. Even if you can remember, you cannot prove it. You can usually remember what you meant—and no one can argue with that.

Compare:

SHE: "I thought you didn't want to take the children with us."
HE: "I'm sorry you thought that. That is not how I felt. I meant that I wasn't sure we could afford to take them with us. I hope we can, and I should know by next week."

The problem is discussed and they are en route to a solution. There is no intervening argument.

Listen to what he or she is telling you *now*. Don't insist on holding onto your past or present impressions. Stop interpreting and pay attention to the literal meaning of what is being said.

Avoiding Arguments

How people talk to one another can be negatively charged and uncomfortable, or warm and expressive. What is said can be badly distorted by *how* it is being expressed.

"I" language enables individuals to express their perceptions without antagonizing each other. Learning to use the "I" language depends on one key principle: Start you sentences with "I": "I would like . . . ," "I feel . . . ," "I need . . ." End them with, "And I'd like to know how you feel, what you would like, what you need."

From there you can discuss and negotiate. Where to go to dinner becomes much easier.

HE: "I would like to have seafood. What would you like to have?"
SHE: "I would like to have steak."
HE: "I know a restaurant where they serve both. Is that all right with you?"
SHE: "Yes, I'd love to go."

Simple, clear, efficient, considerate. Four transactions and the issue is resolved. No conflict.

If you speak from your own point of view instead of in absolutes, communication is much easier. An advantage of "I" language is that, when used correctly, it is very hard to argue. Example: If, when you are in a football stadium, you stand up and announce, "That's the best football game that's ever been played," every fan in the stadium can argue with you. However, if you say, "That's the best football game *I've* ever seen," they have no argument.

Understanding Yourself

Another advantage of "I" language is that you must talk about yourself. In order to do that, you must know how you feel. "I" language forces you to examine your feelings. It also helps you take responsibility for doing something about those feelings by choosing some course of action.

Dropping Your Defenses

"I" language can help you to become more vulnerable, but is that desirable? We build up defenses to avoid getting hurt. (Those defenses rarely work, by the way, and often cause even greater hurt.)

It is not necessary or wise to be vulnerable all the time, even with someone you trust. However, in an intimate relationship, vulnerability is essential sometimes. You need to be able to be yourself, relaxed and at home with someone else in this world. Can you survive without becoming vulnerable? Yes. Are there risks in becoming vulnerable? Of course. If you become vulnerable, you may be in jeopardy (the risk). However, if you are not willing to share your vulnerabilities with someone you are close to, the relationship is in jeopardy. The choice is yours to make.

Eliminating Static

Successful communication requires a sender and a receiver. The message must be clear, must be listened to, and there must be no "static."

What is static? If you are absorbed in a television program, you may not hear when someone talks to you. It won't register, because of the "static." Depending on your point of view, the static can be either the TV program or the conversation.

If you are upset, preoccupied, tired, anxious, worried, angry, or in pain, these conditions and many others will affect your ability to send and receive messages, just as static on the radio obscures music. Recognize and respect the static in your environment. Try to reduce it, or postpone a discussion until the static is gone. Otherwise, you won't accomplish much, and unnecessary arguments often develop.

The following provides a practical guide to help you put these concepts into practice.

Guidelines for Intimate Conversation: How to
Express Your Feelings in Words

---

1. **Start every sentence you speak with the pronoun "I."**
   EXAMPLES: "I'm hungry."
                  "I'm happy."
                  "I'd like to go to a movie."
   It may sound selfish, but it is not. It is clear and honest.
   It is more selfish to make someone guess what you are really thinking. Tell them yourself. "I" language gives someone else information about you.

2. **Avoid starting sentences with any of the following:**
                  "You . . ."
                  "Let's . . ."
                  "We . . ."
                  "I think you . . ."
   "You" is speaking for someone else, and is often accusatory.
   EXAMPLES: "You hurt me."
                  "You are insensitive."
                  "You don't love me."
   Even "You are wonderful" can cause problems for some. ("No, I'm not, you're just saying that.")
   "Let's" and "we" incorporate the other person without consulting them.

"We had a wonderful time." (Maybe she
didn't.)

"Let's go to the play tonight." (Means I want to
go and you'd better come along.)

"I think you" is not "I" language. It only looks like it. You
are talking about the other person, and have disguised it with
an "I think." It is just "you" language in camouflage.

3. **Do not make absolute statements.**

    EXAMPLES: "That is the prettiest girl in the school."

    "That is an ugly dog."

    "That is a stupid game."

Eliminate "that is" statements and substitute "I prefer, I
like, I dislike," etc. People respond to one another and to
their environment through their individual perceptions. It is
risky to impose your perception on someone else through
casual absolute statements.

4. **Avoid asking questions without making your concern clear in
   advance.** "Are you getting hungry yet?" usually means "I'm
   hungry and want to eat soon."

"What's the matter?" usually means "I'm worried that
something is bothering you and need to know if anything is
wrong."

Don't hide your concerns behind a question. Express the
concern and then ask the question.

5. **"I don't know" or "I don't care" are rarely acceptable.** "I
   don't know, but let me think about it" and "I'll tell you as
   soon as I figure it out" are sometimes necessary. You may
   not have *strong* feelings, but you do have *some* feelings. With
   a little effort you can find them. To leave a response at "I
   don't know" is not to have looked far enough for the answer,
   especially if it has to do with yourself, how you are feeling,
   what you would like to do, etc. "I don't care" is inappropriate. When asked "What would you like to do tonight,
   dear?", the response "I don't care" does not actually fit. If
   the response is "How about a snake walk at midnight?",
   you'd suddenly care quite a lot. If you were home alone, you
   wouldn't go to the cupboard blindfolded or select a can of

food at random for dinner. Even if you didn't have much depth of feeling on the matter, you would make a choice. So express a preference even if that preference is not particularly strong.

6. **Do not use "ought," "should," "must," "have to" and similar synonyms.**

SUBSTITUTE INSTEAD: "I might"
                                 "I could"
                                 "I would like to"
                                 "I want to"
                                 "I'd love to"

If you say to yourself "I should get up this morning," and change it to "I would love to keep sleeping but I *want* to get up because I hate being late, and I like my job and want to keep it," it is much easier to get out of bed. But if you can't change it into a "want" because you dislike your work and your standard of living isn't worth the pain, it may be time to give notice. If you can't change a "should" into a "want," reconsider if it is really in your best interest to do it.

7. **Eliminate the word "why" and replace it with "what."** "Why" often comes across as an accusation and puts the other person on the defensive—"Why on earth did you do that?"—especially if they don't really know the answer. Rather than asking someone, "Why are you feeling that way," or "Why are you upset," try, "*What* is bothering you, in *what* way, and *what* might be done to change it."

8. **Eliminate the words "always" and "never."** Substitute "up to now" or "in the past." Human beings are not very accurate predictors of the future. "Always" and "never" encompass the past, present, and future, often resulting in self-fulfilling prophecies. "Up to now" leaves the future uncommitted and acknowledges the possibility of change.

Learning to use "I" language is hard, but not impossible. After a year of conscious effort, it will begin to become second nature. It looks deceptively easy, but it is as challenging and awkward as any foreign language could be in the beginning.

The Misuse of "I" Language

There are pitfalls to "I" language that must be avoided. Determined opponents will argue over it. "You're not using 'I' language!" she accuses. (At that moment, by the way, neither is she.) Don't correct each other. It is easier to see when someone else is not using "I" language than when you yourself are not. Spend your energy concentrating on developing your *own* skills. When tempted to correct someone else, take a closer look at yourself instead.

"I" language is a tool intended to improve communications. Like most tools, it can also be used as a weapon. "I hate you." "I don't like anything about you." "I am tired of you" is technically "I" language. If you add the phrase "right now," those statements are sometimes true just for the moment.

"I" language is an attitude, not just words. It is not an order or a command, but a vehicle for sharing information about yourself, with the understanding that you are interested in hearing the other person's feelings too.

Nothing Is Perfect

Don't let "I" language become yet another belief system. It works most of the time, but not always. It won't work, however, if you are not using it correctly. Determine where the problem lies and fix it if you can. But don't go down tunnel number 4 forever.

When Not to Communicate

The personal growth movement and other extreme I-me philosophies have taken the position that everything should be communicated. If you have an itch, scratch it. If you have a thought, let it all hang out. These schools of thought encourage you to communicate all the time—with everyone. To express every feeling, no matter how trivial, to anyone who happens to be nearby.

Tell the woman passing you on the street that you don't like her hair. Tell your boss what you think of him (or her). If the thought is there, it deserves to be expressed! Not necessarily so.

This method can cause serious problems, including unnecessary relationship crises, and even divorce, when used without judgment and discrimination. Many therapists find themselves trying to patch together a wounded relationship because someone encouraged "Express your anger. Get it all out," or "Be honest about your affair, you'll feel better."

There are times and circumstances when it is better *not* to communicate. If you are tired, premenstrual, irritable, or tense, it is not an ideal time for a serious discussion—especially since you are probably taking yourself far too seriously as it is. Realize that there are some times when you are more vulnerable to an argument than others. Respect those times as much as you can, and don't undertake an important discussion then.

However, don't use this advice as an excuse to go to extremes. Some people never bring up issues at the "wrong" times. That isn't good judgment, it's cowardice. You would face the issue if you could, but you can't so you don't.

Selective communication presumes that you have a choice, that you can participate in a sensible conversation if you wish, and that you can discipline your impulses and defer the issue when appropriate.

Finding Solutions

Often, the use of "I" language makes "right" choices obvious to both. However, after two people have accurately and carefully expressed their respective needs and/or desires to one another there may still be a conflict. This does not necessarily lead to a problem if phase two is instituted: the negotiation of available (and sometimes ridiculous) options.

Most disagreements are kept unrealistically simple: black or white—your way or mine. The argument is limited to two solutions and therefore often goes unresolved, or leaves one person unhappy.

There are usually many options possible, but lack of awareness, inertia, and stubbornness prevent us from exploring them.

For example: The woman wants to go shopping, the man wants to watch "Wide World of Sports" on television. There is only one Sunday to do both. She needs his opinion on something she wants to buy; he doesn't want to go. The obvious options are to stay home (she is resentful) or to go shopping (he is resentful). Less obvious options arise from making a list of alternatives. One of them could be that he stays home to watch TV, while she goes shopping. They both meet their needs, but he feels a little guilty and she feels a little lonely.

Let us look at other alternatives, including a few that border on the ridiculous.

1. She watches the game with him, then they go shopping together.

2. He watches the game, she goes shopping. He joins her after the game to help make selections.

3. They both go shopping. He brings a portable radio with ear plugs to listen to the game as they go along.

4. They both go to the shopping center. He finds a restaurant or bar with TV and watches the game. She shops and consults him periodically, or selects items for his approval during half-time.

5. He records the game if they have a video recorder. They go shopping early. He watches the game with her afterwards.

What is desirable about these solutions is that nobody loses. Both people get their way by cooperating. And sometimes by putting their minds together, they can find an alternative that both of them prefer to their original ideas.

Coming to Terms

When there is an apparent conflict, make a list of all the possible alternatives. She makes a list of alternatives that are desirable *to her*. He makes a list of *his* desirable alternatives. *Do not think of "compromises"*—ways to dilute your preferences to accommodate what you think will be acceptable to the other person. Keep it pure. Then compare your lists and begin considering the alternatives that could suit you both.

It is important to slow down in order to hurry up. Problems crop up and continue because people don't stop to solve them. Because the movie is about to start, or the party is beginning, you forge ahead, without stopping to consider the best course of action.

What is the point of going to a movie or a party angry with one another? Do you really want to endure a strained evening, with an argument as a chaser?

Slow down along the way. Pull over to the side of the road and talk. Solve your differences. Who is running your life? You—or the movie, the party, the football game? Take control and ensure a good time. If a problem develops, stop and address it. Don't let it erode the rest of your day. Take a detour to happiness. It's up to you.

How Long Is Your Lag Time?

There is a lag time for feelings. Most people have it. The lag time is the time elapsed between *experiencing* a feeling and *recognizing* it consciously.

It is important to reduce the lag time. You must be aware of the depth and scope of your feelings *before* making a decision. Afterward is not very helpful. Once you have succeeded in shortening your lag time, the people close to you will understand you better and feel more secure. You will become more effective, as you react to your feelings more promptly, and you will be happier with the decisions you make because they are more apt to be the right ones.

WORDS THAT HURT

This language substitution table is a useful reminder to help you eliminate words and phrases that can get you into arguments, by replacing them with words that are clear, uncharged, and informative.

Instead of		*Substitute*
You, I think you		I feel
Let's		I want
We	"I"	I like
That is		I prefer, etc.

Instead of	*Substitute*
I said	I meant
You said	I heard
Always, never	Up to now, in the past
Should and ought (Synonyms: Must, have to, etc.)	I want, would like, would love, could, might
Why	What
Right/wrong (Synonyms: bad/good, blame/fault)	I like, I don't like

Rewrite or copy this list of words to carry with you for reference, and post in strategic places like the refrigerator and in your office to help you learn "I" language.

Example: You have had a long day at work—your secretary was ill, there were customer complaints all day long, and to make matters worse, you got a traffic ticket on the way home. You are looking forward to walking in the door and just relaxing. Work is behind you. Peace at last.

Your spouse sees the tense, tired look on your face and says: "What is the matter?" "Nothing," you reply. Your spouse insists on probing. Two hours later, you are embroiled in a heated argument.

After it is all over, you realize that although you were coping on the surface, you were in turmoil underneath. Finally, you register the degree of frustration and anger you have been experiencing all along.

When you walked through the door, you were primed for a fight, but you didn't realize it then. The lag time between your feelings and your recognition of them was still in effect.

A feeling can be there for quite a while before you notice it. One patient had a lag time of twenty years. His wife had an affair with his best friend. Twenty years later, when he decided to leave her, he finally realized he had never forgiven her and had been angry all that time.

Remember that the first benefit of "I" language is better communication with yourself. In order to tell someone else how you feel, you must first know your own feelings.

For men, the lag time between their feelings and their knowledge of them is greatest in the emotional zones.

For women, the lag time is most prominent in the sexual sphere. As you practice using the "I" language, the lag time between having a feeling and registering it will decrease, enabling you to express your emotions earlier. Communication will be clearer and more enjoyable. Arguments will disappear from your repertoire, and you will find new solutions to old problems.

CHAPTER 7

Sexual Desire: Her Sex Drive

Sexual desire (libido) is the result of a complex network of influences. The balance of these factors determines the frequency of sexual encounters, and to some degree, the intensity of the experiences.

Hormones influence our sexual appetites. Their exact effect is incompletely understood. Body chemistry has an influence also, as does our state of mind: depression, anxiety, contentment, anger, etc. Genetics and heredity are thought to affect the libido, but we have little evidence to support this yet. It is suspected, but not proven, that sexual scents (pheromones) exist in humans and influence sexual attraction. The current state of illness or health has a bearing as does the degree of fatigue, and whether it is acute or chronic. The quality of the sexual physiological response affects the degree of pleasurable anticipation experienced. In turn, anticipation can be augmented (or diminished) by a partner's response (or lack thereof). An individual's psychological character, in a broader sense, is a significant factor, and is in large measure dependent upon socialization and developmental experiences from earliest childhood.

Let us begin by exploring some of those social and developmental influences.

By the time children become verbal, at age two or three, they know not to talk about sex and not to ask questions about it. They ask questions about absolutely everything else but sex.

Sexual Memories

The earliest sexual experiences that we remember are usually childhood doctor games—you show me yours, I'll show you mine—that occur around the age of four or five. While children often cannot remember any conversation or information about sex prior to that time, they will distinctly remember the adult reactions if they were caught in these experiments. They already knew enough to be secretive and sensed that they were being naughty. (Those who didn't, soon found out.)

One little girl who was showing her brother her genitals and examining his was told by her mother that she had sinned against God, had ruined herself, and would burn in Hell forever after. She grew up thinking that she was physically deformed and would never be able to have babies.

Another brother and sister team were sitting in the family room watching television with their parents. It became obvious to the adults that a rape scene was approaching. In their indecision over whether to turn off the program or not the scene flashed by. Three-year-old Tommy asked, "What is that man doing to that lady, Daddy?" Daddy replied, very uncomfortably, "That man is having intercourse with that girl against her will." "What is intercourse, Daddy?" "That is where the man puts his penis in the woman's vagina." Whereupon Tommy responded brightly, "Oh, I know what that is. Mary and I have tried that too, but my penis is too little and it keeps falling out." At that point, mother and father fell off their chairs, clutched their chests, and regrouped to discuss how to handle the situation. Had they not been as open with their children, they certainly would never have learned about their youngsters' experiments.

Sex is one of the best-kept secrets. When you think of how successfully adults hide sex from children, imagine how resourceful children can be.

Much of our learning stems from role modeling. Where was it? There was none, except to hide sex and any interest in it. As a result, misconceptions about sex abound during childhood.

The Facts of Life and the Easter Bunny

Some young girls and boys conclude that one can get pregnant from kissing; others are convinced that their parents never had intercourse. One of my patients described her reaction when she learned "the truth." She and her nine-year-old girlfriend sat on the curb after church one Sunday discussing this incredible matter, debating whether or not it could possibly be true. They viewed the women coming out of church with a different mind, saying to each other, "Do you think Mr. and Mrs. Jones did it?" "I don't think so, but I *know* Mr. Henry wouldn't do anything like that." "But what about Mrs. Buchanan? She's pregnant, and teaches Sunday School." "You know, I just can't believe it. It couldn't be true." "Do you realize what that means? All the grownups in this congregation who have had children have been doing *that thing* with each other."

Another patient told me that finding out about intercourse was a painful experience for her. When she was just eight years old, her mother told her that it was time she knew the facts of life, and proceeded to tell her about Santa Claus, the Easter Bunny, and intercourse. She was devastated. Her little girl's world was crushed. Now, when she thinks about sex all she can remember is that there is no Easter Bunny.

A girl's moral and religious upbringing usually has a bearing on her later sexual adjustment. Rigid rules and strict parents with a repressive attitude toward sexual matters may result in a woman who does not feel at all comfortable with her own body, her genitals, or her sexuality, who is embarrassed to be seen naked by her husband and undresses in the closet. Sometimes the only way that she is able to respond sexually is by taking the attitude that the part of her that is involved physically is not her real self. By disowning her sensual, physical, and erotic nature, she maintains her self-respect in spite of participating enthusiastically.

Mixed Messages

Young girls are taught not to touch themselves. They are even taught not to wash themselves. It's dark and mysterious down there. It's hard to see, and besides no one really wants to talk about it. Mother (sometimes) washes their genitals carefully for them until they are about three or four and old enough to know what she is doing. After that, if they don't figure it out on their own, no one is going to know. But if you forget to brush your teeth, you're in real trouble. Most little girls don't know how many openings they have, or exactly where they are. The ones who discover their vagina by poking around end up terrifying their mothers who rush them to the doctor's office with a purple discharge, only to discover that three-year-old Debby has put a crayon in her vagina which melted from her body warmth.

Some learn rules, such as don't wear patent leather shoes or the boys might see up your dress in the reflection, and never sit in a boy's lap without placing a magazine there first. One girl concluded that sperm must fly through the air or such preventative measures would not be necessary. Another young lady was severely scolded for coming downstairs to meet the visiting priest without her socks on. She was being improper unless every inch of her skin except her face and hands were covered when she went out.

As a girl matures, she learns it is all right to be romantic but not sexual. She can have romantic daydreams but not erotic fantasies. Even love books and love comics have to be hidden. She is not to be sexual with herself and certainly not with boys. She is told that men will try to get away with what they can, and it is her responsibility to flash the red light and nothing else.

Killing It Early

While woman's sexual interest is influenced by many other factors, the attitudes she is raised with can mold her so profoundly that she ends up with no sexual desire and no ability to respond. The fortunate ones mature to enjoy sex.

Before she is even a teenager, the good girl/bad girl concept has been instilled. Even today in our "modern" society, girls know whose reputations are in jeopardy and how to keep their own intact. There is an image to maintain. Some girls wear ruffles and modest clothing. Others wear low-cut dresses or tight-fitting sweaters.

While socially approved behavior and deportment play a powerful role, specific events in a young girl's development can alter her course. Traumas such as sexual molestation, incest, or rape can have a significant bearing on her sexual adjustment.

These experiences can affect a girl's sexual behavior in various ways. Some blame themselves; they feel they provoked it. Some who have been raised to believe that they must keep themselves pure, conclude that they are ruined and believe that whatever they do from now on doesn't matter. Sometimes they have sex with anyone who asks—not because they enjoy it, but because they see no point in saying no. There is nothing left to protect. Others are so troubled by the experience that they withdraw from any and all future sexual encounters. Touching of any sort, and sex in particular, becomes abhorrent to them.

Eighteen-year-old Cathy came to see me after two weeks of marriage. She was a virgin when she married, and expected that sex would occur naturally. She had no warning to prepare her for her own reactions on her wedding night. At the sight of her husband's penis, she became physically ill. When he attempted to penetrate her, she vomited. Since that day, she had been unable to eat. She lost ten pounds and was developing anorexia nervosa—a serious, sometimes fatal, disorder, characterized by the inability to eat.

No one had told her terrible things about sex during her adolescence. She had never been molested or traumatized in any obvious way. It turned out, however, that to her, sex meant disaster. She came from a strict Catholic family. Her mother, who had been advised for medical reasons to have no more children, became pregnant again. She almost died giving birth, and became an invalid thereafter. Eleven-year-old Cathy was taken out of school to raise her baby brother. She remembers it as "like dying"—being taken away from her friends and her childhood to become an unwilling mother.

A year later, her sister got pregnant out of wedlock, was disowned by her father and forced to leave home. The last news they had of her, she was addicted to heroin and supporting her habit with prostitution.

To Cathy, sex meant pregnancy, and pregnancy in her experience was a disaster. Due to her religious training and strict upbringing, she had not ever experimented beyond holding hands and a brief kiss. Consciously, she did not think of sex as bad. Her emotional reflexes did, however. She was as distressed as her husband that her mind and body refused to cooperate.

Her case is extreme, but it illustrates the point that sex drive is strongly affected by upbringing. Most women's problems are less dramatic, but often no less serious.

For Joan, sex was enjoyable in the beginning, but never compelling enough to interest her if her husband didn't initiate. As the years passed, sex became an inconvenience. She didn't dislike it, but failed to see what everyone made such a fuss about. She wished that it weren't so important to her husband. If it were up to her, she would prefer to live without it. During her pregnancy, it was a relief to have a legitimate excuse to turn him down. She wondered if he was having an affair. She almost wished he would, as long as he didn't tell her about it, so that she wouldn't have to meet all his needs.

Joan is not too different from Cathy, except in the degree of severity, and the fact that Joan doesn't recognize that she has a problem. In her opinion, she is normal. She doesn't realize that the absence of all sexual appetite is not her natural state—that somewhere in her development her sexual desires were so effectively eliminated from her conscious awareness she doesn't even notice their absence.

A Man's Definition of a Nymphomaniac

On the other hand, if a woman is "too" sexual, she may also distress her mate. Kinsey said "A man's definition of a nymphomaniac is any woman who wants sex one more time than he does." Men who are unhappy because their wife's sexual appetite is too low often feel apprehensive when they get what they want, because they can't keep up with her.

There is a great deal of pressure on women to be sexually alive, but demure. Don't threaten men by being too sexual, or by not being sexual enough. Mixed messages again!

The Vagina Has Bad Press

The vagina has very bad press in our culture. And it is no wonder. We're raised to believe that the genitals are dirty. The female structures are not easy to see or to separate in the mind's eye. Sexual hygiene is not usually discussed or demonstrated. Consequently, a little girl becomes self-conscious about her own genitals.

As she grows up, the natural discharges and staining she sees in her underpants worry her, but she asks no one. There are many girls who grow up thinking they have caught a dread disease from the toilet seat. All this fear comes from observing a discharge that is usually quite normal but that no one has ever told them about. Even adult women aren't clearly aware of when a discharge is normal and when it is not. Should there be one? How much? Is there a monthly rhythm to the secretions?

A major reason why some women are sexually reserved or shy is their own discomfort with their vagina. They think it smells bad and looks bad and they feel awkward having anyone touch them.

In a book called *Even Cowgirls Get the Blues* the scenario involved a homosexual tycoon who rose to fame and fortune by developing vaginal hygiene sprays and deodorants to stamp out vaginal odors nationwide. With the proceeds from his products, he built a health spa for women where the classes included detailed odor annihilation procedures with every form of douche and disinfectant imaginable. The cowgirls who ran these ranches rebelled, took over the classes and eliminated the sprays.

Her Sexual Security Number

A woman's insecurity is not limited to her genitals. She yearns to be told she's beautiful, intelligent, and irresistible. She is the willing victim of men who glorify her. "I love you" is the most highly treasured phrase and incredibly readily believed. Most women need outside validation and approval. They don't trust their own judgment sufficiently to feel secure without the constant expressed love and approval of someone they care for.

If Everything Isn't Perfect

A woman's desire is affected by love, warmth, intimacy, and depth of communication. If everything is not emotionally in order for her, sex is not possible. As she grew up, it was romance and love stories that preoccupied her fantasies. Love justified marriage and sex. Sex for sex alone was a nonexistent concept. But add a little love and everything could be there at once.

Atmosphere and Aphrodisiacs

As a matter of fact, for the woman atmosphere alone is often enough. It has an unreasonable effect on many women: candle-light, wine, a fire in a country cabin, moonlight and stars.

"Some Like It Hot"

Other unexpected things draw her out sexually: the helpless man of many misfortunes often attracts her, or the alcoholic who can't get an even break. She is entranced by the sensitive man of promise who needs her help to get to where he'll never be. The impotent man challenges her charms, and she sets her mind to "fixing" him, as did Marilyn Monroe in *Some Like It Hot.*

Diamond in the Rough

Or, the diamond in the rough may appeal to her: the man with a lot of heart and ability hidden somewhere. In the macho man, the big talker, the slightly obnoxious braggart, she sees tender-ness and vulnerability underneath. And then there is the rake who exploits everyone but her. He is putty in her hands. She is his Achilles' heel.

The man who has everything may not attract her. The one with money and looks, poise and position, may have a hard time winning her heart even though he might have access to her body. He isn't pathetic enough; doesn't need her enough. He intimi-dates her with his accomplishments. She may adore him, but feels guilty because she secretly feels that she doesn't deserve him. Her fear that he will leave her, never really be hers, keeps her from making the full emotional commitment she would oth-erwise be free to do.

Sensible Confusion: It's Very Clear to Me

The biological sex drive is there, but the psychological sex drive has its way with her. It can manipulate biological drive in any way it pleases. The psychological drive is vulnerable to all the factors described above. The woman's interest can be most un-predictable, confusing even to herself.

Women usually do know how they feel and feel quite sensible about it. Women who are nonorgasmic can still enjoy sex thoroughly. This is terribly confusing to men. By contrast many women are able to have orgasms, but have no special interest in sex and can live without it.

Biological Urges and Sexual Cycles

We do not yet know a great deal about a woman's biological sexual rhythms, but the evidence suggests that they definitely exist. One survey that studied 3,000 women revealed that about 20 percent of women report no pattern whatsoever to their sexual interest. Another 35 percent identified their time of greatest sexual interest as just before menstruating, and approximately 15 percent just afterwards, which puzzles many rational people. If sex is for reproduction, the greatest interest should be in midcycle, when a women is ovulating. Correct? Wrong. Only 4–6 percent of women said that midcycle was their most erotic time. Two to three percent find themselves sexually ravenous *during* their period, which makes little sense to anyone—especially men. The remaining percentages had more than one time during their cycle when sexual interest peaked.

In this connection, the birth control pill has been studied in depth. Theoretically, if fear of pregnancy was a factor in a woman's sexual disinterest, the birth control pill should be the antidote.

Of the many papers published on the effect of birth control pills on sex drive, approximately 40 percent reported decreased sex drive, 40 percent reported increased sex drive, and 20 percent noticed no change. Women who have decreased libido on the pill are probably the women who have other undesirable side effects from the pill so they don't feel too well in general. Breast tenderness, nausea, vomiting, bloatedness, weight gain, and perhaps depression are sufficient to dissuade them. Unfortunately, none of the studies attempted to correlate these variables.

The 40 percent whose drive goes up may be more secure without fear of pregnancy, or it may be a direct drug effect. There are many unknowns. We know much more about how hormones, blood medications, antihypertension drugs, heart medications, and tranquilizers affect men than how they affect women. It is simpler to study and evaluate sexual response in a man due to his external genital reaction. The woman's pelvic response is more inconvenient to study and more difficult to evaluate. Consequently we have less reliable information about women, and less of it.

Why Nonorgasmic Women Go to Orthopedists

Very few women are aware that their sexual response affects their physical health and their general sense of well-being. One of my referrals was from a frustrated orthopedist who called me saying, "I've examined this woman for her low back pain. There's nothing wrong. She broke down crying in my office and told me all about her sex problems. I didn't know what to do. I told her I was an orthopedist not a psychiatrist. It didn't help."

There is a very good reason that she sought his help. Women who don't function sexually, who are having some difficulty with orgasmic response, or who choose not to masturbate—that is, women who don't have regular sexual tension release—begin to get congestion in the pelvis—the result of blood flowing there. The condition is similar to premenstrual tension, but usually somewhat milder. It may include low back pain and a sense of pelvic heaviness. There is uterine bogginess, and there may be abdominal cramping. The emotional components include irritability, depression, and anxiety. The comment "all she needs is some sex" isn't so far from the truth. This syndrome results from the absence of regular sexual relief.

Making the Connection

If you become irritable or get a stomach ache because you haven't eaten in quite a while, once you recognize the reason for your discomfort you would eat something and feel better. If you don't make this connection, the problem doesn't get resolved. When the sexual connection isn't made, and nothing is done about it, your condition becomes chronic, with associated depression and irritability.

Women often do not recognize the relationship between their mood, their physical well-being, and sex. Thus, nothing is done except perhaps to treat the symptoms with pain pills or back braces. I don't mean to imply that every case of back pain is sexual frustration, so don't go to your orthopedist and tell him that you've had this back problem and now you know what it is. Ask yourself if the occasional backache feels anything like the one that occurs just before your period. If so, you may be experiencing some degree of chronic pelvic congestion.

A Little Physiology: Muscular Contractions

There are four phases to the female sexual response cycle: excitement, plateau, orgasm, and resolution. These phases can be measured in almost any muscle in the body.

During excitement, muscle tension increases—in the arms, the legs, the abdomen, the neck, the uterus. As sexual involvement increases, so does muscle tension. The muscle fiber begins to shorten. The tension increases until plateau levels are reached. The muscle is tense, and it remains tense. The muscle tension that develops is sometimes so intense that it triggers cramps in feet or legs that interfere with the sexual experience, or bring it to a halt before it would otherwise end.

At plateau levels, the muscle ceases to increase in tension. At orgasm, the muscle suddenly contracts forcefully. Once the orgasm has been triggered, several or many contractions may follow. Whether or not a woman progresses to have multiple orgasms, the potential exists for that to happen.

What You Feel and What You Don't

What a person feels is subjective. What actually happens that can be observed or measured by somebody else is objective.

The same objective response can be experienced in two opposite ways. Example: A nonorgasmic sexual experience can be an intense, exciting, pleasurable experience that is exceedingly arousing, very intimate, warm, loving, wonderful, with resolution being a gradual floating down to the base line that you kind of hate to see disappear. On the other hand, that very same experience—that same woman, given a different time, place, and circumstance, can be frustrated instead. "I'm not there yet. What's wrong? Why am I not responding?" with resolution being like fingernails grating on a blackboard.

Many women who have an orgasm don't feel finished. They don't feel done. They feel as if maybe they didn't have the right kind of orgasm, because they are not relieved afterwards. When a woman has one orgasm, even if she doesn't go on to another, since the potential for another orgasm is there, she usually vacillates in plateau for a little while. That vacillation at plateau feeling, where she can go either up or down, is definitely a sense of not being through. She may feel an even stronger sexual urge after one orgasm than when she first got involved.

And then there is that "what's wrong with me" syndrome. And there is nothing wrong. Everything is right. A woman has to be educated about her feelings. Or perhaps uneducated. I think if we had been taught nothing, we would figure it out. But with all the advice we're getting on what to do where, when, and how, it's pretty hard to pay attention to our own body signals—and to react sensibly to them.

A Little More Physiology: The Clitoris

The reactions being described are based on studies done by Masters and Johnson. They observed and measured 350 women in over 7,500 sexual response cycles.

Excitement phase: During a woman's arousal, there are very few noticeable external changes. In the excitement phase, the clitoris enlarges two to three times its usual size. Its sensitivity changes rapidly. A light touch can be too heavy at one moment, and strong pressure might not be enough the next. There is a very fine line between a pleasing touch and an unpleasant one.

Most women prefer a touch that avoids direct contact with the head of the clitoris unless there is generous lubrication. Stimulation to one side or the other, or along the clitoral hood is usually preferred.

Plateau phase: As excitement progresses into the plateau phase, the clitoris shrinks and retracts under its hood. At this time, many women prefer increased pressure, and a more rapid motion.

Orgasmic phase: During orgasm, the clitoris remains hidden and small. In fact, the organ with the most sexual publicity, the only sexual structure with no other function than sexual pleasure, is remarkably small at all times, even when in its enlarged state. Dr. Masters frequently used to comment that it was impossible to know what changes the clitoris underwent during orgasm, because it had never been visible during their laboratory experiments.

As a student, I had the opportunity to observe, along with Dr. Masters, a woman being orgasmic with her clitoris in clear view. As a child, she had had a circumcision—the majority of the hood covering the clitoris had been removed. It was, therefore, impossible for the clitoris to retract under the hood during plateau and orgasm, and we had an opportunity to observe the clitoris throughout the complete sexual reaction. The changes were subtle, but distinct. Initially, the clitoris engorged, enlarged, and flushed with color. At plateau it shriveled, becoming a deep purple. At the moment of orgasm, it became even smaller, almost disappearing from view. It blanched, became pale and colorless. If there were contractions, they were not visible to the naked eye.

The Vagina: Doing More and Enjoying It Less

The vagina reacts more dramatically than the clitoris but feels less. Within ten to twenty seconds of effective sexual stimulation, lubrication begins. A look from someone across a room, a thought, a touch, his hand on yours, can set your body into motion, and you may never be aware that you have lubricated. If the spell is broken, the lubrication will disappear.

Lubrication is an intravaginal phenomenon—a transudate that passes across the vaginal walls. If stimulation is not continued it is reabsorbed by the tissues.

As sexual involvement progresses, the vagina begins to elongate and lubrication continues. At plateau levels, the inner two-thirds of the vagina balloons, while the outer third changes in a fascinating way: it becomes swollen and engorged. Subjectively, this area may become more sensitive than it was before. Masters and Johnson define this zone as the "orgasmic platform." The wall of the inner two-thirds seems to lose feeling while the outer third gains feeling. In actuality, reduced sensation is an illusion. It is just the result of ballooning of the vagina. As the vagina expands, it becomes larger than any penis would ever want to be. The surface of the inner two-thirds of the vagina is usually not in contact with the penis, except perhaps at the deepest part.

Where Is Grafenberg's Spot?

Grafenberg's spot is a zone within the vagina, thought to be particularly sensitive. It is located a few centimeters inside the opening of the vagina, behind the pubic bone, and directly over the tube that leads from the urinary bladder. Stimulation of this area manually, or with thrusting, is reported to trigger orgasms and female ejaculation. If this information is accurate, there may be another circuit for orgasm and the question of "vaginal" orgasms will reemerge. Unfortunately, researchers studying this area have not performed anatomical and histological studies, which would be the simplest way to determine whether or not Grafenberg's spot truly exists as an anatomical structure. Until this research has been done, it is impossible to prove or disprove this new concept.

It is difficult for the woman to touch it herself, but her partner can reach it easily. If you wish to find it, follow these instructions: Lie on your back and part your legs. Have your partner insert his index finger into your vagina, palm facing upward, almost as far in as it will go, curling it upward. Guide him by your sensations. Have him explore until he locates a spot that feels particularly good. *It will not be sensational:* it will be a pleasant, subtle feeling. You may feel discomfort, bladder pressure, and the urge to urinate.

If he finds Grafenberg's spot and massages the area, he may feel a swelling the size of an almond, growing to three or four times that size. You may feel pleasant sensations.

Current investigations suggest that if this spot is stimulated adequately, a woman will become orgasmic—often again and again. These orgasms are associated with a newly defined phenomenon called female ejaculation.

The Cervix Feels More Than We Give It Credit For

The cervix is the opening to the uterus. During menstruation, blood passes through it. For many women, the cervix is a source of sexual stimulation. They enjoy having the cervix jostled with a finger or bumped with the penis. For a few, it is uncomfortable. Be aware of its existence and notice how stimulation affects you.

The Uterus Is More Interesting Than You Think

While the uterus moves and contracts during sex, most women do not feel it. Initially, during arousal, the uterus lifts upward, pulling the roof of the vagina along with it like the center pole of a tent as it is raised. During orgasm, the uterus contracts rhythmically and quite forcefully. The intensity is comparable to the early stages of labor. Those contractions are usually not felt, but are easily measurable using surface electrodes. Just as a few women *don't* feel labor pains, a few women do feel their uterine contractions during orgasm. We do not yet know why contractions are severely painful in one circumstance and undetectable in another.

When the Contractions Don't Stop

Occasionally, a woman will develop some abdominal cramping during or after orgasm. The uterus, which has been naturally contracting during orgasm, goes into cramplike spasm, called uterine tetany. This can be vaguely or intensely uncomfortable when it happens and usually means that there is some minor problem associated with the uterus that makes it irritable and prone to spasm. It is more common after multiple orgasms.

Crossed Signals

Sexual arousal and premenstrual tension imitate each other. Earlier, we described the significant percentage of women who report their highest sexual interest just before their period. The reason for increased libido (sexual drive) premenstrually can be explained on the basis of the pelvic changes during sexual arousal. The responses of the woman's pelvis during sexual excitement are identical to the changes that occur just before menstruation: the increased blood flow to the pelvic organs results in boggy uterus and congested pelvic organs—the same responses that occur during early stages of sexual excitement. The signals get crossed and the messages to the brain are the same.

The forceful contractions of the uterus and the pelvic organs during orgasm recirculate the blood into other areas and the sense of pelvic discomfort is temporarily relieved.

If you are subject to premenstrual tension, try having an orgasm or two (by any method), and see if it makes you feel better. It doesn't work for everyone, but it may work for you.

Biology Moves Her but Psychology Rules Her

The woman's sex drive is intricate—even more complex, it seems, than that of the male. A woman's sex drive is easily decreased. A hurt feeling, an argument, a slight can cancel it for an evening or more. Emotional trauma can eliminate it altogether. Sexual indifference is not usually a natural state.

Her sex drive is not as easily influenced to increase. As women reach their thirties and forties, many notice a stronger interest in sex and a greater capacity to respond. We do not know whether this development is biological or psychological. There are enough women who lose interest in sex as they grow older to confuse the issue. In years to come, we will learn more about her chemistry and hormones. They are unseen but powerful players in her script.

Biology moves her, but psychology rules her. Her aphrodisiacs are touching, gentleness, tenderness, love, intimate talk, atmosphere, and romance. Once her sexual maturity is reached, and the roadblocks and inhibitions of youth are removed, her desire and responsiveness can seem unlimited.

CHAPTER 8

Sexual Desire: His Sex Drive

Most men assume that everybody else is having more intercourse or better sex than they are. Their penis is smaller, or so they think, and they wonder how long they last compared to other men. This kind of self-induced pressure can transform man's natural libido into a competitive event, generating anxiety instead of lust, and feeding an ego instead of a sexual appetite.

Nonverbal Messages

Little boys are taught not to touch their penises. As a matter of fact, Orthodox Jewish males must hold their penis with a tissue or a handkerchief when they urinate to avoid connecting skin with skin. If a little boy is caught playing with his penis, he gets his hand slapped, along with a disapproving "Good grief, how awful" look. He has had erections ever since he was born. Isn't it strange that when Mom began teaching him about his fingers and his nose and his toes, when he was only six weeks old, she didn't say, ". . . and this is your penis." A very obvious structure. It is certainly there. No one has mentioned it yet. He may wonder why, but he doesn't mention it either.

111

Nonverbal messages can be more powerful than the strongest verbal negative message. Nonverbal messages say, "It's too terrible even to talk about." What does the young boy do when he has his first wet dream? He's terrified. No one has told him that it's normal. Is he sick? Is he going to die? Has he got some dread disease from playing with that little five-year-old girl ten years ago? Who can he tell? No one. Who can he ask? No one.

His sexual interest flourishes at a young age and continues to mature. Unlike girls, he is allowed to think sex, and try sex. As a boy grows into manhood, he develops the psychological components of his sex drive. What happens along the way and how he perceives himself will influence his sexual behavior in later years.

By the time a young man has reached the age of puberty he is usually familiar with masturbation. Most boys discover it by themselves, and would patent it if possible. However they avoid "excessive" masturbation. (They usually define excessive as one more time than they do it.)

The boy learning to masturbate soon discovers that the release of sexual tension is also an incredible stress-reduction mechanism. At the same time, he feels guilty and secretive about the process—which increases stress and tension, thus causing more masturbation. In short, he feels guilty, and worries a lot, but it feels too good to stop.

In general, he has had very little sexual education so far— almost none from his mother or father, very little from teachers. Most of his information comes from his peer group.

Adolescent boys learn that it's all right to be sexual and feel sexual—just don't get a girl pregnant, and leave the "good" girls alone. They are also taught that they better figure out how sex works because it's going to be up to them to teach their wives or girlfriends when they get one.

By the time he reaches adolescence, the boy is set on a quest to get sexual experience, but not with girls and not with boys. Very reasonable. Girls are taught not to get any experience at all. Sex is a natural function? Nonsense. You simply don't do it; it isn't proper. Not by yourself—not with anyone else.

Homosexual Experiments and Experiences

Then at age thirteen or so, he begins to learn about homosexuality. While boys are discovering sexual pleasures and are masturbating to erection and ejaculation, they are also beginning to form social contacts with subtle or obvious sexual implications. Homosexual and heterosexual preferences are usually determined during these years. The adolescent youth will usually find out what gives him the most pleasure—and whether that pleasure is with the same sex or the opposite sex.

There is normally some degree of experimenting with the same sex, such as mutual masturbation, self-manipulation with one or more others. (Girls experiment too, but we know much less about the extent of their activities. Each sex usually passes through these phases, and the majority becomes heterosexual.)

A bachelor in his forties came to me for help. He was socially a recluse, impotent, never dated women, and hated the sexual interactions he had with other men. He was a late bloomer, awkward, and timid. He dated a girl once, when he was sixteen. They had ended up necking in the car. When she reached down to touch his penis, he was not erect and she said, "You mean I gave up a date with a real stud for this?" He was so humiliated that he never dated another woman again. He had always felt more at ease with men than with women, but he had no conscious homosexual interest, and remained celibate for many years. He was terrified of women and yet so lonely he decided to experiment with men. In his thirties he had his first homosexual encounter. He continued to have frequent homosexual encounters, but his self-loathing made him seek therapy. He requested help converting to heterosexuality.

While there were other predisposing factors, his pain with women and his contrasting comfort with men had a significant effect on his sexual preference.

The youth who doesn't have the ability or opportunity to date never has the chance to overcome the many fears involved in social contact with the opposite sex. If, by the age of fifteen or sixteen he has had little or no contact socially or sexually with women, he may begin to question his own sexual identity: "I know the reason I'm not going out with girls is because Mom and

Dad won't let me, but I'm not comfortable with them anyway. Could I be abnormal?'' His concept of himself as a sexual and social individual is in severe jeopardy.

Another Male/Female Pattern

It is important to recognize that the sex drives of men and women are affected by different forces. Sometimes the very thing that turns him on, turns her off.

While there are many similarities in the arousal patterns of men and women, the differences that exist often cause considerable problems. He wants her to wear a slinky black thing with crotchless panties—she is horrified. She wants to go dancing or to a romantic movie—he is bored. He brings home a bag of tricks with vibrators and crawling things—she buys twin beds. She wants him to talk to her—he falls asleep. He finally convinces her to see a pornographic film—she gets sick and leaves.

Why is this? Who is right and who is wrong? No one. They are different. A woman wants verbal foreplay. A man wants visual foreplay. She yearns for a setting, a mood, and intimacy (whether she knows him or not). He enjoys legs and breasts. She likes the subtle, genteel, and delicate. He knows sweat and grunts and lust. A woman's physique is visually compelling to him. Men devote special attention to body parts—buttocks, legs, etc.—whereas a woman ordinarily prefers more subtle scenes—a suggestion of sex rather than graphic detail.

A man responds to visual images more strongly than women. He appreciates *Playboy* centerfolds, explicit sexual photographs, adult book stores, X-rated films, and ''raw sex'' to a greater extent than most women do.

Now, there are obviously numerous exceptions to these generalizations, and a great deal of variation among and between the sexes, but these examples illustrate the extremes.

The Squirrel Monkey Experiment

An experiment done with squirrel monkeys demonstrated that the pathway for erection in the male monkey passed through the eye. However the pathway for lubrication in the female did not.

To make this determination, nerves were stimulated at different levels to trace their course. We can only speculate that there are parallels in the human, because no men (or women) have volunteered for the experiments.

Whether the differences are biological or cultural, they are nonetheless differences. The same stimulus won't necessarily affect a woman the same way it does a man.

Fetishes

Fetishes, exhibitionism, and perversions are almost exclusively a male experience. This is not a criticism, but a fact. Women rarely manifest any of these patterns. There are few women flashers, perhaps because they can expose themselves in socially acceptable ways—low-cut dresses and short skirts. Child molesters and rapists are rarely female. Preoccupation with a texture or an object (like a shoe fetish) is also unusual with women. The explanation is not known.

The Madonna Syndrome

The sex drive of some men is affected by pregnancy and motherhood. When a woman becomes a mother, she is no longer seen as a sexual being to them, and their sex drive disappears. Other women will attract them, but not their wives. Affairs are common under these circumstances. This pattern is called the "Madonna syndrome."

This syndrome usually occurs in a man who was raised in the Roman Catholic religion. He personally believes that sex outside of marriage is sinful, but inevitable; sex with his wife is questionable. If she's a good woman, she can't possibly enjoy it and he must be imposing on her. Once she becomes pregnant she is looked upon as a mother rather than as a sexual partner; not as his mother, but as the revered mother of his child. His sexual arousal is replaced by affection, solicitous concern, and tenderness. Erotic emotions are submerged, repressed, or directed elsewhere.

One victim of the Madonna syndrome, feeling desperate, came to me for help. He grew up and lived in Italy. He had a good sex life with his wife until she became pregnant. He could not approach her sexually because she was going to be the mother of his child, so he took a mistress and his life was in order again. This arrangement worked until his mistress became pregnant, at which point he lost all desire for her. He supported his second family like a devoted father and took another mistress, but lived in deadly fear that she would get pregnant. He was afraid that both his money and manhood would run out if this pattern continued.

Not Tonight, Dear, I Have a Headache

Some very sexually active men lose interest in sex after marriage. When a man marries or moves in with a woman, suddenly he has no time off sexually. Both of them expect that he will perform regularly. He has no weekend intermissions, no private time, no place to relax and get away from sexual pressure. Even if the woman isn't pressuring him, he sometimes considers sex a perpetual burden. As a result he begins to withdraw and develops avoidance maneuvers. He fences off intimate encounters that might lead to intercourse. He hasn't learned how to say "Not tonight, dear, I have a headache." He has no way out. The pressure is subtle, subversive, and effective. What he thought he wanted—constant sex, more sex—becomes his albatross. He doesn't want it any more. He feels suffocated and restless without understanding why.

The psychological impact on sex drive can act like a switch, turning on and off with little warning.

A Little Physiology

The sexual response cycle in men (as with women) is divided into four phases: excitement, plateau, orgasm, and resolution.

Excitement phase: The two most prominent genital changes that take place in males during the excitement phase are penile erection and scrotal elevation.

In early phases of arousal, the erection will vary in firmness, whether the owner is aware of it or not. One man reached down to insert his penis and was so shocked to find it was only an "8" instead of a "10" (on a scale of 1 to 10) that he lost it altogether. He then became such a "spectator" that he had problems with erections from then on.

It is hard for a man to tell if the penis is erect without looking at it, touching it, pressing it against something, or feeling it against the fabric of his pants.

Plateau phase: In the plateau phase, the penis becomes as full as it is going to get. There are some color changes of the head of the penis. Shortly before ejaculation, a clear fluid may appear from the tip. It could be a drop or two or quite a bit. This is not a constant feature. Some men have it, some don't.

The testicles enlarge in size by 30 to 60 percent and the scrotum (the sac surrounding the testicles) is elevated, close against the body. Men are not subjectively aware that testicles increase in size at this time. If they were enlarged the same amount by injecting fluid the pain would be intolerable.

During plateau, while the scrotum is fully elevated, a small percentage of men will complain that the testicles will actually leave the scrotum and travel up into their body. This is normal for some men.

Knowing these details of male physiology can make you a more sophisticated critic of pornographic films. The next time you see a sequence in an X-rated movie where the male appears to be ejaculating, notice if the scrotum is hanging there loosely, flopping back and forth. If so, the man cannot be ejaculating—because ejaculation does not take place until the scrotum is fully elevated up against the base of the body. Close-up views in pornographic movies will sometimes show the man's testicles elevated, sometimes low. What you are seeing is a film that has been spliced between orgasms, to combine several separate episodes. The superstuds who seem to thrust forever in those films have actually had several coffee breaks.

Orgasm phase: During the orgasmic phase, the prostate begins to contract, and rhythmic contractions occur throughout structures that propel the ejaculate through the penis. At this point, ejaculation is inevitable and orgasm has begun. It takes a few seconds before the ejaculate actually appears. An internal and external prostatic sphincter (ring-shaped muscle) must work in sequence for ejaculation to occur normally.

The prostate is what the doctor checks with his finger when he examines a man's rectum. It is located below the bladder, and surrounds the tube coming from the bladder that urine passes through. Think of the prostate as an apple with one sphincter at the top and another at the bottom. The upper one must close to prevent urine from being released from the bladder above. The lower one must open so that the ejaculate can be propelled forward. A man who has had a transuretheral prostatectomy—where the center has been cored out of the prostate gland (think again of the apple)—often has a damaged internal (upper) sphincter. This results in ejaculation backwards into the bladder. Men say that the orgasm feels the same way it once did, but no ejaculate comes out of the penis until the next time they urinate.

Resolution phase: During the resolution phase 90 percent of men lose their erection immediately after ejaculation. About 10 percent of men retain their erection following ejaculation and can continue thrusting. The older one is, the more rapidly the erection declines.

The testicles also drop down and shrink in size, returning to their unstimulated state.

The Fine Points of Sexual Physiology

There are two key physiological differences in the sexual responses of men and women. The first is what we call ejaculatory inevitability: that point three to six seconds before orgasm, when the male knows he is going to ejaculate and *there is absolutely nothing that he can do about it.* If the man has passed beyond the period of orgasmic inevitability, a locomotive could roar through the room and he would still ejaculate. The female, on the other hand, can abort her orgasm at any time. This difference can create serious misunderstandings. Women married to men who are premature ejaculators say, "I know he is doing it on purpose because he tells me before he does it.'' In fact, when the man cries out, ''I'm coming,'' it is too late to stop it. She, on the other hand, could stop if she wanted to.

The second major difference is the refractory period: that time following ejaculation before he can ejaculate again. A man, if he is sexually aroused, can be erect again immediately after intercourse—but he won't be able to ejaculate right away. A woman has no refractory period. She can be orgasmic again almost immediately.

Contrary to popular belief, what is biologically possible sexually is not necessarily desirable. The ability to be multiorgasmic can be compared to the ability to have extra helpings at dinner. Sometimes you want to and sometimes you don't. You rarely eat as much as you biologically could because it would feel uncomfortable. Then sometimes it's grand to be a glutton.

I don't become erect immediately after ejaculation as you say men can. Why not?

Men don't inevitably become reerect. They can, however. Some do and some don't. The most significant determining factor is interest. If a man becomes reinvolved and reinterested, he's very likely to become erect again. Since so many males are under the misconception that once they have an orgasm they won't be able to become erect again for a certain period of time, they don't even try. It doesn't occur to them, so they never discover that they can. Many men, after ejaculation, get drowsy, sleepy, and uninterested in further sexual activity.

After they have had an orgasm or two, women are often ready to cuddle—at least—and continue at best. They may still be experiencing plateau phase and consequently the mood of the moment is to stay involved.

Why is there a time difference in the refractory period with intercourse? One time my husband will ejaculate the second time after fifteen minutes of rest; another time it takes hours.

Refractory periods will differ from time to time, from situation to situation, and from male to male. The man who was able to have the most number of ejaculations in a laboratory situation had three within a ten-minute period. That is unusual, however. The average refractory period for most teenage boys is ten to fifteen minutes. In one's twenties, thirties, and forties it may be half an hour or more. Factors that influence the refractory period are:

- Number of immediately previous ejaculations
- Age
- Fatigue
- Alcohol
- Drugs
- Interest

In one situation it may be ten minutes, next time it will be two hours and it continues to vary throughout. Age is definitely a factor: the refractory period that was ten minutes at age sixteen may be three days at ninety.

Testosterone

Testosterone is a male hormone that is liberated in greater quantities at the time of puberty. It is what makes men "masculine." It causes their voices to be deeper and hair to grow on their face. It causes them to become bald, to get larger muscles than females, and to get coarser hair on their arms and legs. Baby boys have testosterone too, but at puberty there is a surge.

Once sexual behavior has been activated and learned, it seems to remain fairly constant regardless of changing testosterone levels. Eunuchs were popular centuries ago. Young choir boys were castrated (had their testicles removed) to keep their voices high and beautiful. Eunuchs were also used to guard harems in Arabic countries.

If a boy was castrated before puberty, and had never had the opportunity to learn sexual behavior, he never became erect and never developed libido. Since he did not develop large muscles, he was not really desirable as a harem guard. So, harem guards were generally castrated after puberty as young adults. These men were already sexually experienced. They were not castrated to keep them from having sexual intercourse, but so they couldn't make the females pregnant.

Contrary to popular belief, once a man has learned how to function sexually, even with removal of his testicles, some can continue to have intercourse. However, there is no doubt that his sex drive declines.

Castration in our society is sometimes done for medical reasons, such as in treating cancer of the prostate or testicles. Often that man's libido has already decreased due to ill health, and it is difficult to gather good research data on this subject. There is as yet no reliable information to show how testosterone alters the male libido. I see many men in therapy who have very high testosterone levels and low libidos. Some men with low testosterone levels have high libidos.

Testosterone has a seasonal and diurnal variation. A man's early evening level is about 25 percent of his 8 A.M. level. Therefore, the blood test should be done in the morning to check the highest levels. Testosterone levels are highest in September and October. They are lowest in April. The significance of these seasonal differences is not understood.

Your Biggest Sexual Organ

Physical signs of sexual activity also occur in other areas of the body—and are just as important to the ultimate sexual response as what takes place in the pelvis. Keep in mind that your biggest sexual organ is your skin. Depending on your frame of mind, and who is doing it, wherever you are touched can be arousing.

Chemical Help

Attempts to understand chemical and hormonal effects on sex drive have not yet yielded consistent or meaningful results. It is clear, however, that these influences exist, even though their nature has not been fully determined.

There are drugs with properties that selectively decrease libido, such as cardiac medicines, certain tranquilizers, megase (an antitestosterone medicine), and DES (diethylistilbesterol), which has been used effectively to control impulses of sex offenders. There is no doubt that specific drugs that selectively increase sex drive will soon be discovered. Several drugs are currently under study, some of which are discussed in Chapter 14.

The normal libido varies greatly from person to person, causing stress for couples who are on opposite ends of the spectrum. Will it be possible someday to install a chemical rheostat in a man or a woman, by giving titrated doses of a medication to increase or decrease sex drive? Until then differing sex drives will continue to challenge the sexual integrity of a relationship.

Men and women are biologically, psychologically, emotionally, and chemically different. Their disparate sexual drives get them in more difficulty with each other than almost anything else. Differences in their sex drives are to be expected. However, once interested, contrary to popular belief, both men and women can become aroused equally intensely and almost instantly.

These differences do not inevitably lead to problems, but they often do. The Totaled Woman, whom you are about to meet, is a typical example of what happens when sex drives cause conflict.

CHAPTER 9

The Totaled Woman

About those women (and men) who avoid sex

Why Do Women Who Used to Enjoy Sex End Up Dreading It?

The Totaled Woman once enjoyed sex, now she is too tired. She used to pursue it (no matter how subtly), now she turns away. Other men appeal to her, but not her husband. Or, she openly dislikes sex and would prefer to live without it. She is often depressed, has low self-esteem, and is aversive to sex. The sexual troika is running away with her. She is on the brink of a severe personal crisis that can destroy her relationship.

DEAR ABBY: Thank you from the bottom of my heart for publishing all those letters from women who admitted that they didn't enjoy sex all that much. I thought maybe there was something wrong with me until I heard that lots of women felt the same way.

I raised four children (all married now), and my husband and I have really had a good marriage. But as far as sex is concerned, I have been living a lie for 25 years. I have never really enjoyed sex, but I have learned to fake it so well, believe it or not, my husband thinks I'm over-sexed.

NO NAME, PLEASE

123

DEAR NO NAME: According to my mail, if all the women who deserve an Academy Award for convincing performances were placed end to end, they'd reach Masters and Johnson's in St. Louis.

The erosion of a woman's sensual desires takes place over a period of many months or years. Along the way, she gains what she thought was much sought after, recognition—as Superwife and Supermom—and also becomes a gracious "Lady in Waiting."

Superwife and Supermom

Almost every woman tries to become one or both. Some try harder than others. Consider the woman who goes to work when she has young children because it is an economic necessity. She is determined to show the world she is not falling short in any of her responsibilities at home. To prove this beyond the shadow of a doubt, she overcompensates to the point of exhaustion.

She works at a paying job from 8 A.M. to 5 P.M. In her "spare" time she fixes meals, gets the children off to school, shops, cleans, cooks, chauffeurs, cheers at Little League games, always looks good, and is available for sex whenever her husband wants her. She tries to be the Perfect Wife described in Chapter 1.

When the world isn't looking, she complains bitterly, is chronically tired, depressed, resentful, and occasionally suicidal. She is so guilty that she can't take even a few minutes to relax without feeling she ought to be doing something else— like scrubbing the floor. A vicious cycle sets in that sabotages her self-esteem and puts sex on a back burner—sometimes indefinitely.

The Lady in Waiting

While Superwife was working diligently to live up to all of her own, her mother's, and her husband's expectations of what a wife ought to be, and Supermom was beginning to get bedraggled, the Lady in Waiting is aging gracefully. She is constantly postponing the things that are important to her in life until some future time or event: "When my husband finishes school, my kids grow up, we get more money . . . I will go back to school, start my career, take art lessons . . ."

After a period of years (it seems like a lifetime) of trying to be Superwife, Supermom, and being a Lady in Waiting with nothing happening, she begins to wonder if anything ever will.

Latent Aversives

Most women have been subjected to the Superwoman concept to some extent. Consequently, probably any woman is, under certain circumstances, susceptible to becoming aversive. That is why the problem is so common.

Men susceptible to aversion are often the kindest, gentlest individuals at heart. They are also usually perfectionists with high expectations of their sexual performance.

Among women, some are more prone to aversion than others. The classical "good girl," who is programmed to be very dependant on the approval of others, is especially vulnerable.

Women learn at a young age that boys don't marry girls who have sex. "You are not to get into bed with anyone even if you are in love with them (but only then)." She also learns that love and sex are inseparable: "If he really loves you, he won't have sex with you." However, "Only have sex with someone you love." Is that clear? I didn't think so.

When the "good girl" first settles into marriage, things go well for awhile, sexually and emotionally. However, no matter how well motivated she is to always be sexually available, there are times when she really does have a headache, or is not feeling well; times when she is depressed or upset; times when she is very angry with her husband and doesn't feel like sex; times when she can't stand the sight of him.

"I Gave You the Best Years of My Life"

Her sense of invulnerability has faltered, her denial system is crumbling. Her hope for the future is grim.

DEFINITION OF TERMS

SEXUAL AVERSION is a sexual dysfunction characterized by the *continuous* avoidance of intercourse, as well
as any touching or physical intimacy that might lead to
sex. The aversive male or female may find the sexual
experience unpleasant, or be orgasmic and enjoy it.
Even the ones who enjoy it will still generally avoid sex.
Aversion occurs primarily in committed relationships.

THE AVERSION REFLEX is an involuntary negative
emotional response to sex or the anticipation of sex.
This reflex develops when sex becomes psychologically
or physically painful for an extended period of time. Its
mild form involves vague uneasiness related to sexual
advances by a partner. In its severe form, an affectionate touch by a spouse or lover can generate emotional
panic and acute anxiety.

LATENT AVERSIVES have poor self-esteem and a large
capacity for guilt and resentment. They have been
taught that a good wife never says "no" to her husband
sexually and a good husband is obligated to satisfy his
wife whenever she is in the mood. When exposed to a
sexually stressful situation (such as rape, difficulty having orgasms, impotence, or an aversion carrier), they
readily develop sexual aversion.

AVERSION CARRIERS are men or women whose sexual
satisfaction is inordinately dependent upon their partner's responsiveness. They are displeased, critical, or
hurt if their partner is not sufficiently aroused and they
use guilt as a powerful tool. "You don't satisfy my
needs, you're an inadequate sexual partner, you spend
too much money," etc. The aversion carrier is critical,
complaining, demanding, and never satisfied. The aversive partner feels under constant pressure to perform,
and is blamed for their unsatisfactory sex life as well as
anything else that goes wrong.

1. Her husband is not succeeding in his work as they expected he would. He is not measuring up to her expectations—or perhaps is excelling instead and leaving her behind.

2. There is financial insecurity, with young children, house payments, and impossible budgeting.

3. Marital problems have surfaced. She doesn't see her husband very much. He's busy working to support them all, and is constantly running away from her complaints at home.

4. The children wear her out. They are good kids, just normal, average kids. "How did my mother ever manage with six?" she wonders.

5. School, college, and work have passed her by. She suspects getting married was a big, irrevocable mistake.

6. She has little sex. She doesn't want much more, actually, because she is too tired. Nonetheless, she realizes that there should be more to love and life than she has.

7. She is disappointed in many things, confused, unclear why she is so unhappy when she should be on top of the world.

8. She finds herself chronically angry and resentful—when she is not depressed—and blames the children, her husband, and life in general for her miseries.

9. She succumbs to the "I gave you the best years of my life" syndrome. "My unhappiness is all your fault. If it weren't for you . . ."

10. She may have an extramarital relationship in her search for the comfort and love she feels can no longer be found at home.

11. Her physical fitness has deteriorated and she has become anxious about her appearance. A sense of desperation creeps in: opportunities are over, she is too old to find another love.

12. She undergoes tremendous upheaval in her value systems, challenging all that she has been taught to believe, and resenting her parents and a society that pressured her into an early marriage.

Do You Feel Guilty When You Say No and
Resentful When You Say Yes?

As angry as she may be with her husband, these circumstances can still produce guilt feelings. "It's my fault, I shouldn't deprive him." Eventually, instead of having sex with her husband because she wants to, she gives in whenever she feels guilty enough: "It's been a week . . . He really has been patient. I wouldn't blame him if he went looking for someone else . . ." So, she has intercourse because her guilt index is up. Then she goes through the motions instead of the emotions.

Immediately after the sex, she gets resentful because she said yes when she didn't want to. She feels that he took advantage of her (although she agreed and went ahead). She remains angry until her guilt index starts rising again.

This guilt/resentment syndrome is usually time-related. Each woman has her own particular rhythm. For some women it's a day, for others a week, or a month. For some it's a year before she feels guilty enough to have sex. At some point the guilt reflex is triggered and then it's "yes." Afterwards, resentment sets in and it is "no." Sexual frequency is determined by guilt and resentment instead of sexual ardor.

The No-Win Situation

This woman is in a no-win situation, a double-bind in which she has no psychologically comfortable way out. If she says yes, she'll feel resentful and if she says no she'll feel guilty. Either way, she loses. Sex becomes a chore, and she starts avoiding it.

Her husband is also in a no-win situation. If he approaches her and she agrees, he feels he is imposing on her. If she rejects him, he feels deprived.

The Aversion Reflex

The aversion reflex is a powerful emotional "no" that sets in whenever her husband approaches her. Once affectionate, she now can't bear to be hugged, touched, or patted—except in public. There, she feels safe because it won't lead to the bedroom.

She can't say no with comfort (although she usually says no these days) and she can't say yes with comfort (although she capitulates sometimes). She develops various avoidance maneuvers—some more direct than others—so that she is not forced to make an unpleasant choice.

Avoiding Him

She takes a new tack, and becomes very busy. She may decide to go back to school, and will probably have classes that meet when her husband would normally be home, or she may get deeply involved in community affairs. I am not suggesting that she does this knowingly or maliciously; or even that she understands what is motivating her. She is desperate to bring separation between herself and her difficulties. All activity-prone women are not aversive, however, so do not make any hasty diagnoses.

Common aversion maneuvers can include: different bedtimes, reading late at night, saving all the housework for when he walks in the door, being always "too tired," crowded schedules, business worries, long hours, alcohol, fatigue, relatives and friends always underfoot or living in. Be suspicious of arguments that occur regularly before bedtime if sex has become a stressful situation. After the argument starts she is safe. He will be too angry to suggest sex.

By this time, sexual aversion is well established, but most couples do nothing about it.

Male Aversion

Men become aversive too. In fact, impotence is often the result of an underlying sexual aversion. Sex has become a chore, so the man avoids it; it takes so long for her to be orgasmic (or perhaps she never is) that he prefers not to get involved; or he gets discouraged and bored during sex and so does his erection. The impotence isn't medical, it is due to anxiety or fear; it is the result of sexual aversion. Sometimes, a man who had a strong sex drive before marriage changes overnight.

Suddenly my husband doesn't want sex. When I try to discuss it he will not communicate. He says: "I don't need that kind of life anymore, I'm indifferent to sex." What has happened?

Sexual aversion, though less frequent in males than females, is usually more severe. As noted above, it results when sex has become psychologically or physically painful in some way. If sex becomes work, an *A*-to-*Z* project, he tends to avoid it. Even when he might feel like a little sex, he won't pursue it if he thinks it means a tense, hour-long session, or if she always complains that he ejaculates too soon, or if no matter how hard he tries she doesn't have an orgasm.

A man whose wife cannot reach orgasm may get aversive because he feels it's his job to satisfy her and his failure if he doesn't. Every time he confronts a sexual situation, he is also confronting his own personal failure. It is not that he has such a big ego, or that he is such a fragile person; it's just that he cares. Her lack of responsiveness convinces him that he is doing something wrong.

When problems like this last for a long time without a solution, sexual aversion is almost inevitable. It begins with a loss of interest. The libido is canceled by negative apprehension. Any persistent sexual problems—either his or hers—can cause aversion in the man, just as impotence in the man can cause aversion in the woman.

As he reaches a certain age, the man can say the same thing as the menopausal woman: "I'm off the hook, I don't have to face this anymore."

Celibacy

A person who is sexually aversive is not the same as a celibate even though the end result—lack of sexual activity—may be the same.

A celibate is a person who voluntarily avoids sex for a specific reason, religious, moral or ideological. This is a conscious choice.

Aversion is rarely the result of a deliberate decision. Rather, it is usually a subconscious reaction to an inability to enjoy sex for physiological or psychological reasons or to a dread of that inability itself.

How Can You Tell If You Have Sexual Aversion?

Sexual aversion, as we defined it in the beginning of this chapter, is the continuous avoidance of sexual activity.

1. There is an apparent or real difference in sexual appetite. The spouse who feels rejected usually increases sexual advances, which only drives the partner farther and farther away. If either of you has said, "All she (he) ever wants is sex" or "She (he) is never interested in sex," assume sexual aversion is present until proven otherwise.

2. There is an absence or decrease in casual touching. Affection is rarely expressed with physical gestures.

3. The aversion reflex sets in, and there is tension over a touch, a hug, or a kiss. Both of you end up irritated, upset, or angry when a sexual approach is made.

4. Avoidance maneuvers develop to provide convenient obstacles to intimacy.

5. Sexual frequency is reduced to two times a month or less. The only sex drive left operating is the biological urge. The psychological desire is gone. If aversion is severe enough, it will even cancel the biological urge, and result in no sex at all.

6. Aversion doesn't usually occur until commitment develops. The husband often feels betrayed or tricked, especially if aversion occurs shortly after marriage. He doesn't realize that it is happening, in part because she cares so much.

7. Love becomes an issue and escalates the crisis. He accuses her of not loving him because she doesn't want sex with him. She accuses him of not loving her because he is insensitive to her feelings.

8. There are two different types of aversion: the man or woman who once enjoyed sex, but no longer does; and the person who has never liked it. Their patterns differ.

The woman or man who has become aversive within the relationship, but found sex pleasurable once upon a time, is usually aversive *only* to their mate. Affairs are common, and usually enjoyable, sometimes developing into a second marriage. Once commitment occurs, however, aversion develops again. Ironically, he or she often enjoys sex (even with the committed partner) once actually participating, but avoids it as much as possible anyway. There may be no other serious sexual problems, but some will develop eventually if the aversion persists. This type of aversion is more common in women than in men, and responds very well to sex therapy.

By contrast, the person who has been aversive all of his or her life is usually aversive to *all* members of the opposite sex, not just the spouse. These individuals rarely have affairs. There is almost always another specific sexual problem present: impotence, premature ejaculation, absence of orgasm, and vaginismus (defined in Chapter 13) are the most common. They rarely enjoy sex during the experience, and usually actively dislike it. This form of aversion is more common among men, and is somewhat more difficult to treat, because it is often associated with other emotional problems.

Aversion Is Catching

If one person is aversive, and consequently avoids sex most of the time, the other person eventually avoids the opportunity to be repeatedly rejected. He or she will no longer try to initiate sex, because of the predictable negative response. Thus the aversion has spread. But an even more serious consequence is that when both people are aversive, they rarely seek therapy. They do not want any help to get them more sex when they can no longer stand it and would prefer less.

Earlier Is Better

There is only one thing nice about the Totaled Woman syndrome: this woman gets so miserable so fast that she tends to wake up a lot earlier than most men do. (Men usually aren't aware of the extent of their discontent until their forties or fifties.) It is a very difficult time for her and those who love her. She knows that she is unhappy—in fact, she is miserable.

The Totaled Woman knows what she doesn't want, but not what she does want. That is a terrible dilemma, because what she doesn't want is usually everything she has. To set new goals feels like an almost impossible task. She may spend several years giving her husband a terrible time—being irritable, complaining, demanding. She becomes absolutely horrible to be around and hates herself more and more every minute, saying, "Look what you've made me into, I was not like this until I married you." Her husband can't understand what has happened to the wonderful young woman who used to be so easy to get along with.

Taking Command

Gradually, painfully, she realizes she must stop being a Lady in Waiting and decides that "the only one who is going to make me happy is me." She starts that difficult process of learning what she wants, what will make her happy, and deciding that she is worth it. For the first time she starts taking risks. Her desperation can be measured by her radical decisions. She has an affair, her husband finds out. She leaves her husband and children. Six months later she wants him back and he's gone. However, from that point on, her growth process—although still filled with pitfalls—becomes more fun. She has a sense of finding out "who I am, what I want," and she is willing to take the risks to do something about it even though she may make mistakes. She still has difficulty taking risks, but she grits her teeth and takes the chance.

However, it is not necessary, or desirable, to make such radical changes. Sexual aversion can be cured without destroying the relationship, without divorce, without open warfare.

Once the problem is recognized and understood, it is possible to rehabilitate the relationship, eliminate sexual aversion, and not just mend fences, but make that marriage stronger and better than it ever was.

Small changes in several areas are far more effective than sweeping changes in one.

Don't Let Sex Fall Apart Too

As these problems manifest themselves, sex tends to fall apart too. The woman feels that the very fact her husband would want sex is an insult, "because he knows I don't like sex when I'm angry. If he wants to have sex when I'm angry, then he doesn't care about me. He's not treating me like a person. He disregards my feelings!" Things go from bad to worse.

A woman must learn to have sex not to service her husband or to satisfy him, but because it feels good to be close, because she knows she cares for him and they like one another—and because there's something in it for her. At that point, an upward spiral develops and there's a place to buffer the problems that occur in other areas.

When there are sexual difficulties, who says you can't still be nice to each other? If the man is a premature ejaculator or the wife isn't having orgasms that is trouble enough.

How to Keep Your Sexual Pilot Light Burning

Considering that it helps to be psychologically ready for sex, how do you make that mental switch when you've had a very busy day, all kinds of things are going on in your head, and yet your husband comes home and wants to jump into bed before you get dinner on the table?

It is difficult for most women to handle this situation because sexual thoughts are surprisingly absent from women's minds. It is not just an issue of being too frazzled to have sex on your mind right at the moment. It is a matter of not thinking about sex often enough to make the time for it in your life. You just fit sex in, rather than plan it.

The reason women squeeze sex into otherwise full agendas is because all those years of conditioning not to think about sex were so successful!

What makes you hungry? Sometimes it's signals from your stomach, but usually, it's your mind: the smell of food, reading a menu, making your supermarket list, just thinking about last week's dinner party can make you hungry. By the same token, a sexual fantasy is thinking about sex, looking at sex, building it into your thoughts, dwelling on something you find sexually erotic. Make sex a part of you rather than keeping it in some secret compartment. How many times have you been made hungry by food elsewhere, but gone home to your own kitchen? You needn't worry that allowing yourself erotic thoughts and feelings means that you will become promiscuous.

Sharpen your sexual appetite. Become more aware of your sexual feelings—drag them out from time to time just so that you can act on them later, whenever you choose. If all your sexual energies are turned off, all pilot lights shut down until the big event, it may be impossible to kindle even a tiny flame. Put another way: If the electricity is down, you may not be able to get your generator started. Keep a sexual pilot light on.

If women would cultivate their sexual thoughts and erotic interests—allowing themselves to look, think, and feel—their sexual inertia could be overcome.

How can sex help you to remain friends despite difficult times? Why do some couples have this ability while others don't?

The way to remain sexual friends when things are rough is to turn toward one another and hold on tight. When you are the most furious, and just can't stand the sight of the rat, put your arms around him and hold him close. Right now that sounds easy to do, but at the moment of fury it is a gut-wrenching struggle.

Say to yourself: "I am absolutely furious with him right now, but I know I care for him and I wish we were getting along better. Since nothing else is working, and we're just getting into more deep trouble, I'm going to get as physically close to him as I can."

The first time is the hardest. The second time isn't all that easy, but the third and fourth times you do it, it starts to make sense—because it works. You'll find that it is awfully hard to stay mad at someone you are holding close (even if that person stands there rigidly with their hands in their pockets and their lips tucked in between their teeth because they are mad at you too).

If the two of you have talked about this remedy ahead of time and said: "I think holding will help, let's both try to cooperate," then when one person makes the gesture the other will probably make every conceivable effort to respond. When I say "respond" I don't necessarily mean to hug back and be actively loving, but to be accepting as opposed to rejecting. There will be times when one person is too upset to interact, but more often than not it will work.

If two people who are not getting anywhere by other methods start to touch and hug affectionately and perhaps to have sex, the whole atmosphere changes. An example: You've been talking for three hours. You still don't understand her. She's absolutely furious with you. You're both exhausted. She can't figure out how to say it again, or why you don't understand. You are not too fond of her at the moment either. Talking for a few more hours isn't going to do you any good; neither is going to bed feeling hostile toward each other. If you say, "Hey, I'm not getting anywhere except upset. I'd like to go to bed and hold you for a while," you'll be amazed at what that can do for your tattered, stressed, tense psyches.

Another factor may also be operating. When you're hungry, you're irritable and very likely to fight with somebody. When you haven't had sex in a while, there are the psychological and physiological effects of no sexual tension release lately. That leads to a heightened sense of irritability, anger, and greater tendency toward depression. Consequently, when people are having the most difficulty, and when they're feeling low, sexual tension release could be the best solution for both of them.

The Risk of Divorce

While some sexual problems can be tolerated almost indefinitely, aversion often leads to a rapid divorce. And the main reason is not sexual at all: the issue is "love." Tragically, each partner feels unloved and rejected. The fact is, nothing could be farther from the truth: if the love and commitment weren't there, the problem would not have developed in the first place. However, the intensity of the pain and the feelings of rejection can become unbearable.

Aversion rarely goes away by itself. In fact, if untreated, it becomes progressively more severe. However, for couples who enter therapy instead of court, the prognosis for success (substantiated with hundreds of cases) is excellent, if the therapist is experienced in treating sexual aversion.

Reversing Aversion

When you are really turned off to sex but love your spouse, how can you turn back on without the resentment?

It is very difficult, especially without some kind of help, but it can be done. Begin by reflecting on the origins of resentment. Resentment comes from holding somebody else responsible for your unhappiness. You cannot successfully resent someone for having intercourse with you if you recognize that they couldn't do it without your cooperation—no matter how passive, sluggish, or resistant you may feel inside. Whatever is going wrong has occurred with either your passive or active cooperation.

A passive decision is just as real a decision as an active one. If you reach over and hold someone's hand, who is holding whose hand? As long as there is no glue and no handcuffs, the other person has the opportunity to withdraw his hand. If the individual chooses to leave it there, he is holding your hand too. It doesn't matter who initiated the action.

While both men and women can become aversive, it is more commonly a feminine manifestation of sexual troubles. The following pointers on reversing aversion are often directed to women, but can be helpful to men who are trying to cope with similar problems.

Start having sex for *you,* too. If you go into sex with the attitude that you are just a service organization, or are giving in to him, there is no way for it to be enjoyable—much less fun. Approach sex with the attitude that you want to enjoy the experience. That does not mean an "I'm going to get my orgasm if it kills me—or him" approach. Instead, say to yourself, "Rather than using all my energy resenting him, I'm going to have a good time."

When a woman believes that every time she has intercourse she is *giving somebody a gift, and losing something of herself,* that is harmful.

You must participate, not "give." Unsuppressed *participation is the best gift.* If you have fun sexually by doing something for yourself he will probably love it too. Don't be a Lady in Waiting—waiting for someone else to figure out what to do. It is time to stop thinking, "I wish I had more of this," or "I wish he'd do that," and to start saying "Here's what I'm in the mood for tonight, how about you?" If he is not interested in that suggestion, begin touching him in a way *you* enjoy. Don't give him a massage—that's work—unless you love the way it feels to massage him. Stop gearing all your efforts to pleasing him. Please yourself and you will do both. Otherwise you will continue to be haunted by your resentments.

When you think you are doing things for him, it is usually an illusion, anyway. You are doing them for yourself, but just don't realize it and blame him instead. Think of all those times you had intercourse to please him or because he "pressured" you. It must have been easier to give in than to say no. You would rather have sex than live with the guilt or have a disagreement.

Your greatest ammunition against resentment is self-responsibility. Put that into practice and you will be impressed with the change.

If (based on the information in this chapter) you feel that you are experiencing sexual aversion, you are already en route to increased insight and understanding of one another. Recognize that you are in the grip of a conditioned reflex. Stop the arguments about who does or doesn't love whom and consider the fact that you most probably love each other in spite of the apparent sexual disinterest. If necessary, live as brother and sister for a while. Become friends again. Don't expect to understand one another's feelings completely, but listen and talk. Once you realize that you are both on the same side, the battle dissolves and your energies can be used to improve your relationship.

For the Totaled Woman, especially, sex begins with a gentle word. She is sensitive, insecure, and quick to feel criticized. No matter how hard she tries, she cannot learn to enjoy sex for someone else. When she decides to explore sex for her own pleasure—to discover what she enjoys—and educate her partner to her preferences, she opens the door to change.

If you are unable to reestablish your friendship or, in spite of doing so, the quality and frequency of sex do not improve within a few months, it is time to consider professional help.

CHAPTER 10

The Orgasm

A Simple, Accurate Picture of a Woman's Orgasm

Many books and articles have been written about the woman's orgasm. There is so much contradictory information in print that no other subject in the field of human sexuality has people so confused.

NEW MYTHS ARE REPLACING OLD MYTHS

OLD MYTH: Women should have one orgasm—if any.

NEW MYTH: If a woman doesn't have multiple orgasms each time, something is dreadfully wrong.

FACT: In the past, women were taught not to show their sexual feelings. They are now being pressured by men, and by themselves, to have more and more orgasms. A woman usually doesn't feel like having a climax with every sexual experience. It's not that she can't, sometimes she prefers not to. At times she will want several. At other times she may not want any.

OLD MYTH: It isn't terribly important for a woman to have orgasms.

NEW MYTH: Female orgasm is a glorious experience that changes a woman's life.

FACT: The quality of the sexual experience determines its value and importance in a woman's life, not just the orgasm. There are women who have orgasms, but hate sex. There are women who have never had an orgasm, but love sex. If a woman has an unsatisfactory sexual relationship, even becoming orgasmic is usually not enough.

139

OLD MYTH: Vaginal orgasms are superior to clitoral orgasms.

NEW MYTH: Clitoral orgasms are superior to vaginal orgasms.

FACT: Both orgasms feel good. However, they are different from one another in intensity and quality, depending on time, interest, and circumstances. One method of stimulation isn't better or more mature than another. Each woman has individual preferences, which will change from time to time.

OLD MYTH: Manual manipulation is cheating.

NEW MYTH: The considerate lover always massages the clitoris during intercourse.

FACT: Manual manipulation before, during, or after intercourse is not cheating. When a woman has an orgasm, who is to say what triggers her response? When two people are thrusting vigorously, it may be a kiss, a thought, or another touch that causes her orgasm. Manual manipulation is appropriate and considerate whenever it feels good. However, during thrusting it can be distracting for the woman; and uncomfortable for the man, whose hand is sometimes twisted into an awkward position and wedged between two bodies.

OLD MYTH: There is no way you can tell if a woman is having an orgasm.

NEW MYTH: You can tell if a woman is being orgasmic by nipple erection.

FACT: Nipple erection usually occurs during orgasm, but not always. Nipple erection also occurs when a woman is chilled. There is no way a man can tell between the two, unless he asks her and she tells him!

OLD MYTH: Love is essential to satisfying sex.

NEW MYTH: Love is irrelevant to sex. Technique and a sense of fun are everything.

FACT: Love and sex occur separately as well as together. Your sex life can be better if you are in love. Sometimes love makes sex worse (see Chapter 9). Sex without love can be fabulous, or traumatic. In general, a healthy person with the capacity to love can also enjoy sex without love.

Whose Orgasm Are You Having Now?

Freud informed us that there are two kinds of orgasm: clitoral and vaginal. He concluded that the vaginal orgasm was the "mature" one, and that the clitoral orgasm was "immature," and therefore inferior. This concept drove many women into therapy, with the desire of becoming more sexually mature.

Kinsey's 1953 survey of sexual response concluded that approximately 60 percent of women were orgasmic with intercourse.

Shere Hite's questionnaire survey of women for her book *The Hite Report* concludes that only 40 percent of women are orgasmic with thrusting. Figures from a Redbook survey of about 100,000 women are higher. Since the experts still disagree on the percentage of women who are orgasmic with intercourse, the figures available remain suggestive, but not conclusive.

Masters and Johnson, who clinically observed, researched, and documented sexual activity in the human being, state that *physiologically* there is only one type of orgasm.

In 1979 Whipple and Perry described a category of women who ejaculate during orgasm through stimulation of a special area inside the vagina called Grafenberg's spot. They suggest it must involve nerve pathways different from the type of orgasm described by Masters and Johnson. For a more detailed description, refer to Chapter 7.

Recent research on female sexuality has produced great public interest in a subject not even discussed in private ten years ago. While there is a great deal of information available, there is still much we do not know about human sexual responsiveness. It is important to understand clearly what is known, but it is equally important to be receptive to new discoveries as they develop. This chapter will sort fact from fiction, provide a useful understanding of orgasm, and offer guidance on how to interpret the continuing onslaught of new information about orgasm.

How Many Types of Orgasms Are There?

The most commonly asked question about orgasm, after "How can I learn to have one in ten words or less?" is: "How many kinds of orgasms are there?"

Depending on what source you read, you will discover that there are: vaginal orgasms, clitoral orgasms, blended orgasms, uterine orgasms, mixed orgasms, mutual orgasms, mature orgasms, immature orgasms, multiple orgasms, ejaculatory orgasms, terminal orgasms, the right kind of orgasms, and the wrong kind of orgasms.

Are there two different kinds of orgasm, vaginal and clitoral, or is there only one kind? I have read that all orgasms are alike and that women experience no difference between vaginal and clitoral orgasms.

As far as we know, there is basically one biological type of orgasm. However, all orgasms don't feel alike any more than all itches and sneezes feel alike. The physiology is the same, the organs involved are the same, but the event that causes the orgasm will vary, and the feeling that results can be different in quality and intensity.

If we categorized orgasms based on the method of stimulation used, the list would begin with vaginal and clitoral, but we would have to include other methods: fantasy orgasms, small of the back orgasms, big toe orgasms, rope climbing orgasms, nipple orgasms, etc . . . for there have been women able to have orgasms in these ways and many more.

Clitoral and vaginal stimulation are the most usual methods. A majority of women are able to be orgasmic with clitoral stimulation. Many are not able to be orgasmic with thrusting alone.

The "Perfect" Orgasm

There is confusion about what orgasms should feel like, how many to have, and when to have them.

A common misconception developed from unrealistic expectations causes some women to be disappointed when they don't feel like this: the romance is exquisite, your feelings race against your will. You lose all reason, becoming an animal, wanting just One Thing. Finally, the explosion, the bells, the fireworks. (The earth may tremble.) Then all of the blood runs out of your head and you faint. Paralyzed, you lay there spent, exhausted, and content.

Many modern novels perpetuate this myth, but what women actually experience is quite different. These false expectations lead to unrealistic goals and create sexual problems that would otherwise not exist. Many women who are quite normal mistakenly think they have a sexual problem because they do not react like the women in *True Romance*. They sometimes resort to faking orgasms in a desperate effort to appear normal.

The Terminal Orgasm

A woman patient once asked me how she could have a terminal orgasm. She was not feeling suicidal. She simply wanted to have an orgasm just like her husband's—one that was so strong that she would collapse afterwards and be unable to move. The French call this typically male reaction *petite mort* (little death).

Wonder Woman

There used to be three clear-cut groups of women: those who had orgasms, those who did not, and those who did not know what they were. A fourth group is now emerging. I refer to them as Wonder Women. These women know that there are such things as orgasms, and wonder whether or not they have ever experienced one. They are not sure. They read avidly about sex. They talk to other women (but not about themselves), hoping someone will drop a hint that will finally make clear to them exactly what an orgasm feels like. In the meantime, they continue to wonder whether *that feeling* is actually an orgasm, or merely a preview of the "coming attraction."

How can a woman know if she has had an orgasm or not?

Most orgasms are recognizable without too much difficulty. However, some women doubt if they are really having orgasms because: they don't feel worn out afterwards; they are often left wanting more; the feeling at the time wasn't very strong or distinct.

An orgasm can be a quiet Mother's Day, or an explosive Fourth of July. How it feels is not measured by physical intensity alone.

If you suspect you are being orgasmic, you probably are. Some women have a series of low-intensity orgasms with intercourse, sensations that are not as pronounced as those they experience with self-stimulation. Often, after a woman has had an orgasm, she feels like continuing. Her capacity to be multiorgasmic, even if she never actually is, can keep her sexual momentum going and give her that unfinished feeling.

What Is an Orgasm?

Let's see if we can sum up exactly what we do know about orgasm to date.

Physiologically: According to the extensive research of Masters and Johnson there is only one type of orgasm. There is only one nerve circuit set into operation, regardless of the source of stimulation. If nerves or circuits are missing, a woman will not be orgasmic by any method. If her system is intact, she has the potential to be orgasmic in a variety of ways. For example, it is well known that men have nocturnal emissions (wet dreams) in their sleep. These experiences are mechanically the same as the erection and orgasm a man has when having sex. If he is able to have wet dreams, he has the physiological capacity to ejaculate. His sexual wires are hooked together correctly.

By the same reasoning, if a woman is orgasmic in a sleep state, or if she has ever been orgasmic in a waking state (with or without a partner), we know that she has the physiological capacity to be orgasmic. There may be psychological roadblocks and barriers to her ability to be orgasmic, but her body is working. The necessary raw material with which to work is present. So, if a woman can be orgasmic *in any way,* no matter how unusual or how bizzare, she is physiologically capable and has the potential to be orgasmic in other ways, too. There are new theories emerging about a two-nerve circuit, but the data is still inconclusive.

Intensity: The intensity of orgasm varies according to the method of stimulation involved. While there are many individual exceptions, in general, an orgasm with a vibrator is far more intense than an orgasm with manual self-stimulation, and an orgasm with manual manipulation by partner is more intense than an orgasm with thrusting. Intensity also varies with mood, frequency, and cycle.

Psychologically, orgasms do differ. Although for most women the orgasm with intercourse is the least intense from a physical standpoint, it is psychologically the most enjoyable and satisfying. Orgasms attained with masturbation or with a vibrator are the most physically intense, but psychologically and subjectively the least satisfying. The key is how they are perceived.

Masters and Johnson conducted a study in which they asked women to rate the intensity of their orgasms on a scale of one to four, one being the least intense and four the most intense. In another room, a physiologist who did not know which method of stimulation the woman was using, recorded the intensity of the orgasm the woman experienced. Afterward, each woman's response was compared to the physiologist's rating. Although neither knew the number given by the other, the results consistently agreed.

The women reported the opposite of what had been previously believed. Orgasm with self-stimulation was rated at three to four. Orgasm with partner stimulation was rated as two to three. Orgasm with intercourse was rated as one to two.

The women were then asked to rate the three methods of having an orgasm a second time, based on which they enjoyed the most. The rating was reversed: they enjoyed orgasm with intercourse the most in spite of the fact that it was the least intense and orgasm with masturbation the least even though it was the most intense.

Since the time of the study by Masters and Johnson, vibrators have come into common use. Although women rate vibrator orgasm as the most intense of all, they rarely if ever elope with them. Physical intensity isn't everything.

While women do not become addicted to vibrators, it sometimes becomes their only method. It is usually so quick and easy that many women lose patience with other forms of stimulation. There are some women who have had their first orgasm using a vibrator and have not learned to be orgasmic in other ways. This is not addiction, and an improvement on having no orgasms at all.

Methods: Some women have been able to be orgasmic just by rubbing the small of their back or simply using fantasy—the "look, Ma, no hands" approach. These, too, are "real" orgasms. Only the method of stimulation is different. Some other methods by which women have become orgasmic are: performing oral sex on their partner, nipple stimulation alone, listening to the noise of an airplane flying overhead or the sound of car engines. Orgasm while listening to music or dancing also occurs. A patient came to me for treatment because she could be orgasmic only through fantasy; if her husband touched her she became distracted and lost all sexual sensation. The list goes on.

How do you know if a problem is physical or mental?

If you can have orgasms by one method, but not another (i.e., with self-stimulation but not with partner manipulation), the problem is almost always mental. If there is pain or discomfort, the trouble is usually physical. Occasionally, mental problems cause pain with intercourse, but more often, pain with intercourse causes mental problems.

How many orgasms should a woman have?

As many or as few as she wants. Some women are capable of having dozens of orgasms in a row. In a study to determine the most orgasms a woman could have, it was discovered that one woman could have 100 over a period of thirty minutes to two hours. That doesn't mean she preferred that many, any more than someone who wins an egg-eating contest wants twenty eggs for breakfast.

Sexual appetite varies from person to person, and in the same person from day to day. Sex should be treated like any other natural function. The number of orgasms a woman has should be determined by the urge, desire, and feeling of the moment; not by her partner, a sex manual, or someone else's theory.

The Orgasm

What actually happens to a woman's body while she is having an orgasm?

What follows is a detailed description of the physical responses that occur during orgasm. Some occur all of the time; all of them occur some of the time.

As most men know, orgasm is a total body response. Women sometimes fail to recognize that during orgasm almost every body system is involved to some degree. Your breathing increases, sometimes to the point of hyperventilation, and you are probably perspiring. The major muscle bundles in your body, in your thighs, pelvis, buttocks, and arms, are forcefully contracting and relaxing. Your hands go through a grabbing motion. Your feet stretch or strain downward. Your back is arched. Your head is tossing. You may moan, gasp, pant, or even scream. Your face does not have the serene, content, soft smile you may have seen in the movies. It is tense, grimacing, strained, and distorted.

If someone took a picture of your face during orgasm, and didn't know what was happening, it might look like you were in great pain.

The pelvis undergoes changes too. The outer third of the vagina contracts rhythmically; so does your rectum. The clitoris remains shrunken and hidden under the clitoral hood and does nothing spectacular. There are no visibly interesting changes in the external genitals other than in the percentage of women who may ejaculate some clear fluid from the bladder opening. Internally, the uterus, which is the size of a small fist, contracts forcefully.

Does a woman ejaculate?

Recent studies suggest that some, if not all, women may ejaculate during orgasm. It is thought that a fluid (not urine) comes from the urethra (opening to bladder). A problem in interpreting what actually happens is that some women do pass urine during orgasm. These same women also usually pass small amounts of urine when they laugh, cough, sneeze, dance, or jog.

It appears that female ejaculation during orgasm does occur in at least some women. Current research will undoubtedly provide more conclusive information within the next few years.

In an effort to identify the source of the fluid, women have been given a pill that dyes their urine blue. The fluid from an "ejaculation" is collected, analyzed, and compared to urine, by color and chemical composition. The color was significantly lighter than the blue of the urine. Preliminary studies have found the composition of the fluid *not* to be urine, but to resemble the prostatic fluid of the male.

Do women ejaculate? Possibly. If so, do all women ejaculate, or just a certain few? In spite of the recent book, *The G Spot,* we still do not know.

Uterine Contractions

Some fascinating procedures were done to determine what happened to the uterus during orgasm. If sex was indeed for reproduction, the uterus must have sucking contractions to pull the sperm up into the tubes for fertilization. If the contractions were expulsive instead, they seemed to be meaningless and counter-reproductive.

When the original conclusions were published showing that the contractions were expulsive, they provoked such an uproar that Dr. Masters performed additional studies to refine his data. First, he studied women during orgasm under a special kind of X-ray equipment. A cap filled with dye that would show up on X-ray was placed over the cervix (the opening to the uterus). If, during orgasm, the dye was sucked into the uterus, it would show on the X-ray and demonstrate that the uterine contractions were sucking in nature. In fact, none of the dye was found in the uterus during or after orgasm.

In a second study, he had women stimulate themselves with a doctor's metal speculum in place so that he could watch what happened to the cervix during orgasm. All of the women studied were having their period. If the contractions were expulsive, it was felt, blood would be forced from the uterus and would be observed coming out of the cervix. As it turned out, the uterine contractions were so forceful that blood was expelled from the vagina, splattering the white lab coat Dr. Masters was wearing.

These are the physiological reactions that women experience during moments of orgasm. Some women have only one orgasm at a time; others have many. A few women have one long one that doesn't stop until the man does. (This unusually long orgasm that continues until all stimulation stops is called a status orgasmus. It is rare.)

Multiple Orgasms

Women have the potential to have more than one orgasm. They can have several orgasms in a row, without stopping. Multiple orgasms can be measured as a cluster of uterine contractions (three to eight) interrupted briefly, and repeated at intervals. Some women define multiple orgasms as more than one orgasm occurring during the same sexual encounter, even if the orgasms occur at one-hour intervals. Most, however, consider these individual orgasms and define multiple orgasms as those occurring in rapid succession (within seconds or two to three minutes).

After the first few orgasms, the intensity of each response generally diminishes. In between orgasms, a woman's clitoris might become momentarily hypersensitive, before being able to continue stimulation. The capacity to be multiorgasmic is delightful for most women, with peaks of orgasmic tension occurring in rapid succession until stimulation is stopped, or until satisfaction or exhaustion terminates the experience.

Is That All There Is?

After a woman has had one orgasm, she may have an unfinished feeling. This occurs because she is capable of having more, and she remains at plateau levels of sexual tension for a while. Even if she does not go on to have another orgasm, she usually remains sexually interested, feels emotionally high or personally intimate, and often likes to cuddle, talk, and continue touching.

Deluged by a plethora of incorrect information about orgasm, women have developed unrealistic expectations. They often feel that the orgasms they are having are not worth all the fuss made over them. The experience is nice, of course, and feels good; the woman loves experiencing orgasms and would miss not having them. But, it isn't that spectacular and she can go from day to day without longing for another one. In other words, expectations so far outstrip the reality that women ask themselves, "Is that all there is? Am I missing something? Am I having the right kind of orgasm? Is this the best I can do?"

"Doctor, My Vagina Is Numb"

A similar complaint among women who come in for help is "Doctor, what's wrong with me? My vagina is numb." It's only numb by comparison to their expectations. Of course they feel something. They feel warmth, pressure, friction, and moistness. When expectations are so far removed from reality, a woman is not apt to even notice the feelings she does have. She does not take the opportunity to build on those feelings, enjoy them, and foster their growth into more intense feelings. When her mate is a conspirator in trying to identify what is "wrong," they both begin on a quest of pursuing her abnormalities instead of her sexuality.

If You Have Never Had an Orgasm

If you have never had an orgasm, you have no frame of reference for how one feels. Or do you? Many women who consider themselves nonorgasmic have indeed had orgasms. Do you mean that you have never had an orgasm under any circumstance to the best of your memory? Or do you mean that you have had orgasms in some ways, but not with intercourse? If you have had an orgasm under any circumstances, in a sleep state, as a young girl, or by some usual, unusual or unexpected method, you have had the subjective experience of what an orgasm is. You are not "nonorgasmic."

On the other hand, you may very well fall into the category mentioned earlier: Wonder Woman. A number of women who come to me for therapy describe themselves as nonorgasmic. After a few visits, some of them begin to realize that the "mild sexual feelings" they have been having with intercourse are actually low-intensity orgasms. The more attention they focus on enjoying those feelings, the more distinct those orgasms become.

Stop Competing

The woman who stops comparing her own feelings to everything she has been told she *should* feel, and begins enjoying the feelings she *is* having, will notice that the feelings get stronger and stronger. Eventually, they are quite recognizable. As long as she stays busy ignoring them, judging them, or comparing them to someone else's feelings, they are prevented from getting more intense. The more attention she focuses on enjoying her feelings, the more distinct those orgasms become. Instead of trying to measure up to some arbitrary standard, stop competing.

If you are still in doubt, take a pencil and paper and describe in detail your most intense erotic experience. The words won't come easily. However, do so before reading on, then compare what you have written to the material that follows. What conclusions do you draw?

Were you aware of any mild pulsing sensations or throbbing in the vagina at the peak of the experience? Was there a flush of warmth in the pelvis or across your chest that seemed to come in waves? Did your muscles tense up? How much? Was there any air being forced into or out of your vagina at the peak of the experience? The answers to some of these questions can help you to reevaluate whether you are being orgasmic or not.

Then ask yourself the following questions: How did you feel afterwards? Have you been expecting to feel exhausted, drained and totally content? If so, you are misleading yourself. Perhaps you may have incorrectly concluded that you are not being orgasmic based on your expectations of how you should feel afterwards.

If a woman never has orgasms, is it physically harmful?

Not as far as we know. Being what we call anorgasmic (or nonorgasmic) does not cause death or any serious medical problems. However, mild chronic problems such as the pelvic congestion syndrome discussed in Chapter 7 do often result.

Should You Believe What You Read about Orgasm?

No, not without subjecting the information to careful scrutiny. It is hard to evaluate what you read about a subject as mixed with emotion, biology, love, and fear as sex. How do you know what is based on good, responsible research and what is based on someone's theory, fantasy, or wishful thinking? Here are some guidelines to help you identify reliable information.

The first step is your attitude. Don't believe everything you read. Take away the Ph.D., the M.D., or whatever title the author of the material you are reading has after his or her name. Then read the material as though your neighbor wrote it. Apply your common sense to the information. Does it stand on its own? If it doesn't sound very credible coming from your next door neighbor, the odds are it isn't credible from anybody else either.

Don't assume that you are abnormal. It is too easy to allow your own inferiority complex to cloud your judgment. Assume, instead, that you are normal until proven otherwise and read the material from that point of view. Then bounce the information off of your own experience. Ask yourself, Is that how I feel? Is that how I respond? Does that happen to me? If the answer is yes, then you know the author is at least partially on target. If the answer is no, be skeptical. The range of what is "normal" varies tremendously. It is tempting to see oneself as abnormal, due to fears of inadequacy, but don't mislead yourself. Information is a powerful tool that can make your life better and improve attitudes and circumstances. However, it can also do the opposite if you give it power over you by believing everything you read.

So, be a good consumer. You compare prices when shopping, you look for the best buy, and are suspicious of too great a bargain. Be just as conscientious in evaluating the material you store in your mind.

What We Don't Know about Orgasms

There are some important questions for which we do not have the answers. We don't know, for example, exactly how hormones or other chemicals affect a woman's orgasmic capacity. We don't know why some women are easily orgasmic and why some have great difficulty; or if there are genetic or familial sexual patterns that continue for generations. If your mother, your grandmother, and your sisters are not orgasmic, does that mean that you can never have an orgasm, and if so, is it the consequence of the way you were raised or of a hereditary trait? We also don't know the neurological pathways for orgasm. We don't know if women ejaculate during orgasm and where the fluid comes from, and we don't yet know the anatomy or the significance of Grafenberg's spot.

Most of all, we don't know how to say we don't know, and that is why so much incomplete and inaccurate information is passed as truth from generation to generation. Trends and fads in sexuality are misleading.

Some surveys today indicate that fewer and fewer women are actually orgasmic with intercourse. Is this true? As time goes on, are women becoming less sexually responsive? Or, are they perhaps becoming more open, accurate, and honest in talking about themselves?

There is no way to be certain, but given both the current statistics available in research and impressions from my clinical practice, it appears that estimates of the percentage of women who have orgasms with intercourse are lower than formerly believed, and estimates of the number of women being orgasmic through masturbation and other methods involving clitoral stimulation are probably not high enough.

Do You Really Want to Be Normal?

It takes courage to look inside oneself and attempt to answer one's own questions. To do so means giving up the quest to be normal; for the quest to be normal causes people to repeatedly fall victim to myths. Women, unfortunately, continue to be rather easily programmable in both their expectations and in their responses. The history of sexual patterns demonstrates that when women are told that it's improper to react, they lie still and restrain or conceal their responses, desperately wanting to be normal. Then, later, when they are told it's abnormal not to have orgasms, they make every effort to do so and seek therapy if they cannot.

The definition of normal, in most cases, is very arbitrary, *and changes*. Accepting someone else's values and outside definitions of normal without questions can be harmful to your mental health.

Modern Orgasms

Today's trend is for women to have many orgasms. Mutual orgasms are not as popular as they once were. Tomorrow, if you don't ejaculate, you will probably be considered deficient.

I don't suppose an orgasm today is too different from one a hundred years ago or one a hundred years from now. The only thing that is changing is our professional analysis of them. I can't think of a better way to make a woman feel inadequate than to make her believe she isn't having the right kind of orgasm, or enough of them.

Until we know more, much more, women must trust their own responses and consider themselves normal until proven otherwise.

We do know that most women who have never had an orgasm can be taught how to have one, that if a woman would like to become orgasmic with intercourse she can usually learn to do so and that women are capable of being multiorgasmic.

There are methods of becoming orgasmic that tend to work reliably well. Following the recommendations in the next chapter can help you to become orgasmic if you are not, and to enjoy sex more if you are.

CHAPTER 11

How to Have an Orgasm Whether You Want One or Not

A Sexual Recipe for Women (That Men Need to Know About Too)

The biological, psychological, and emotional aspects of orgasms have been described in Chapter 10. This chapter will focus primarily on methods of becoming orgasmic. For those who are already able to have orgasms, the suggestions to follow will increase the intensity of your orgasms, the speed of your responsiveness, and the variety of methods by which you can experience orgasm.

What Is Normal?

It depends on what authority you read, and in what decade. Small wonder then, that women have become confused. Even the normal ones think there's something wrong with them: their vagina is numb, their orgasms take too long, or their climax is not the kind they want to have.

The "experts," unfortunately, continue to generate fear and insecurity by creating problems that wouldn't exist without them. These sexual trend setters decide on a new definition of normal, and create instant problems to cure. Just add water and mix.

Common sense gets lost in the quest for supersex. But hold your ground. Remember that if you can have an orgasm by any method at all, your body is wired together correctly and you are physiologically intact. That is normal! If a new "expert" decides next year that the real way to have an orgasm is by finger-to-ear stimulation, that will not suddenly classify you as abnormal, unless you allow it to.

It is possible, however, to have orgasms in new and different ways if you are so inclined—not because there is something wrong with you if you don't, but to add to your pleasure. If there is a way that you would prefer, that you think would be more fun and make you happy, by all means apply the suggestions in this chapter and see what you can learn on your own. If necessary, get a little additional help through therapy.

How often should I be orgasmic?

Don't expect one every time. Most women are orgasmic 40 to 80 percent of the time, by one method or another.

What method should I use?

Whichever method you enjoy.

How long should I take to have an orgasm?

The time will vary. If you are getting sore or tired, it is taking too long. If you are getting anxious or frustrated, you are probably pushing yourself too hard. A reasonable range is from ten to twenty minutes. (Some women can be orgasmic within thirty seconds.) That does not mean that half an hour or forty-five minutes is too long. If you are deeply involved and thoroughly enjoying sex, you'll stretch the experience out as long as possible, sometimes hours. However, if you require thirty minutes to an hour every time, it may produce a great deal of stress and strain. If your children won't leave you alone for that long, or if business and social engagements crowd in on your time, sex can become a chore. ("We've got fifteen minutes, dear. Hurry!")

What Kinds of Problems Are There?

The most common complaints among women are that it takes too long to achieve orgasm or that they can't reach a climax with thrusting alone. A large number of women worry about their partner getting bored because they take so long. Or they are concerned because just as they are beginning to become involved, their partner ejaculates. They are left aroused and unsatisfied. This frustration leads them to seek help.

Most women come to a therapist to find out if they can reach orgasm in a different way. Some women can reach orgasm by one method and not another; or perhaps several methods work, but not the one they would prefer to use. There are women who are orgasmic only with self-stimulation; others are able to be orgasmic under some circumstances and not others. One woman came to me as a patient because she could only be orgasmic with intercourse. Her husband was impotent due to diabetes. She needed sexual release, but didn't want to leave him or have an affair, so it was very important to her to learn to be orgasmic with partner stimulation and masturbation. Some women who have orgasms without difficulty would like to become multiorgasmic. A somewhat extreme case was that of a patient who discovered that she could have an orgasm while sitting on her washing machine during the spin cycle. It was the only way she could achieve an orgasm. Her goal was to learn to be orgasmic with her husband.

Suppose you simply can't have orgasms. Does that mean you are frigid?

Definitely not. Most women who do not have orgasms are easily aroused, warm, loving, and enjoy sex. They simply don't happen to have orgasms. The absence of orgasm for some women does not detract from enjoyment as much as men, and to some extent women, have been led to believe. Orgasms are very nice to have, but it is not necessarily a disaster when they are missing.

My wife has been doing a great deal of reading about sex recently. She has never had an orgasm, and blames it on me. I now seem to have lost interest in sex. Why?

Some women feel very angry about not having orgasms. They feel cheated and treated unfairly by a life that has deprived them of orgasms. Their anger focuses on men whom they feel, in retrospect, have all exploited them. They accuse their present partner of being insensitive, inconsiderate, uncaring, and selfish. They are usually too angry and indignant to be nice, and consequently it is often difficult for a man to feel sexual toward them.

Thinking You Have a Problem Can Be One

One patient consulted me for the following problem: every time she became aroused, her body tensed and became quite rigid. Fearing that she had a terrible mental block about sex, she saw a psychiatrist. After five years of psychoanalysis, there was no improvement, and she decided to see a sex therapist.

This woman was absolutely normal. She had no problem except her belief that she had a problem. The tensing of her body was a natural sexual development. She was told to encourage it, rather than resist it, and reached orgasm the very next time she and her husband had sex.

If you think you have a problem, that alone is problem enough, and must be taken seriously. A man who thinks he is a premature ejaculator (whether he is or not) can worry himself into impotence. A woman who thinks she should have orgasms with intercourse every time will feel inadequate even if she often has orgasms with intercourse.

Unrealistic goals and unmet expectations bring some women into therapy. Some expect to feel more than is biologically possi-

---

THE TYPES OF PROBLEMS WITH ORGASM

The following circumstances generally, but not always, create problems in a couple's sex life.

1. Orgasm with self-stimulation only, requiring an object of some sort; such as a vibrator, running water, or hairbrush.

2. Orgasm with self-stimulation only, requiring a limiting, unusual, or uncomfortable position, such as legs tightly held together, lying on stomach, rubbing against a door knob, climbing a pole, etc.

3. Orgasms with self-stimulation and partner manipulation but not with thrusting.

4. Orgasms with thrusting but not self-stimulation or partner stimulation.

5. Orgasms which happen very infrequently, regardless of the method of stimulation.

6. No orgasms at all under any circumstances.

ble. Others want to have mutual, multiple orgasms with every encounter. Possible, perhaps, but not probable.

Preparing Your Mind

Your mind is the most significant sexual organ you have. It is more powerful than any mere physical technique. Therefore, preparing your mind is the most important prerequisite to a fulfilling sexual experience.

If your mind is filled with anxieties, fears, resentments, distractions, and frustrations, you will not feel sexual. Unless you can clear out these unpleasant feelings and substitute thoughts that have erotic meaning for you, you will not become aroused no matter what you do physically.

First, you must have peace of mind. See that you will not be interrupted. Ensure privacy.

A variety of specific techniques—mental techniques, not sex techniques—are discussed in the pages that follow. Read them carefully and have fun applying them.

The Fishbowl Concept: Mental Techniques

Think of your mind as a goldfish bowl that can only hold so much. If it's full of fantasy and erotic thoughts, you'll begin feeling sexual. If even a little "mindspace" is taken up by "I wonder if Janie is going to burst in on us," or "His hand must be getting tired," or, "I wonder what I should serve for dinner tonight," the fantasy and sexual feelings can be crowded out.

We tend to think of our minds as having infinite capacity. True, the mind is magical and marvelous, but at any given moment it can only register a limited amount. A fishbowl, after all, can only hold so much.

Fill the fishbowl of your mind with erotic thoughts and feelings before a sexual encounter begins. Otherwise you will usually not feel "in the mood." Being in the mood for sex will usually not happen to you out of thin air. Nor is it your man's sworn duty to provide it for you at any given moment. You must make the effort to generate the mood in order to become pleasantly receptive to a sexual encounter. There are many ways to fill your fishbowl. None are successful all of the time, but most of them are effective most of the time.

FANTASY.   One way is to choose a pleasant sexual fantasy and focus your thoughts on it. For example, think about the last or best sexual experience you have had. Remember the details—how you felt, what you did. If you dwell on a particular fantasy enthusiastically you'll find that it enables you to shift gears from routine day-to-day living to degrees of sexual transport that will enable you to increase your potential responsiveness. Perhaps you'll want to visualize a tropical island, a warm sandy beach, and a full moon. Or perhaps some slow dancing in your living room, with candles burning and a fire crackling in the fireplace.

If your mind is having a good time, lost in erotic wanderings, savoring the excitement of the moment, your body will probably follow in those same tracks. So, let the daydreams flow on. If you're toting up the week's grocery list in your head, chances are you won't even lubricate.

Many women say they don't or can't fantasize, but that is usually untrue. If you think you can't fantasize, think back to when you were a teenager and used to daydream about being a beauty queen, or falling in love with Rock Hudson, Clark Gable, or Cary Grant. Remember fantasizing the hugging, the kissing, the romance? That is fantasizing. Just take it a little further.

If you are completely stumped and feel you can't fantasize at all, get a copy of Nancy Friday's *My Secret Garden* and borrow a few of her fantasies.

I feel guilty if I fantasize anyone else but my husband. Should I fantasize only about him?

If you only fantasize about the man you are with at the moment, that is not fantasy. That is reality. The ability to imagine sexual experiences with other people is one way to prevent monogamy from becoming monotony. Fantasy is not the same as wishful thinking. You may enjoy in fantasy what you wouldn't consider in reality. Sometimes fantasy is wishful thinking. A man may fantasize oral sex and want it, too. At another time he may be having intercourse, fantasizing oral sex, and enjoying them both at the same time.

I have rape fantasies and sometimes imagine I am a little girl who is being seduced by an older man. Is there something wrong with me?

If using that fantasy is the only way you can become aroused, there is something wrong. However, most women have rape fantasies, and they are quite normal. If you ask a woman: "Do you really want to be raped?" she will say, "Of course not. He may be ugly, rough, have bad breath, or hurt me. In fantasies I can orchestrate everything. I am in control. I definitely do not want to be raped in real life." Her fantasy is not wishful thinking. It is enjoyable only as a fantasy.

THREE EROTIC THOUGHTS. If you find that sex is rarely on your mind (even when you are having it), try the following technique:

Have three erotic thoughts a day. It won't happen without your making a conscious effort, so you will have to remind yourself frequently.

Remember, the thought must be erotic *to you* or it won't help. Thinking of animal sex doesn't count if the idea disgusts you. A few examples of erotic thoughts are:

- A silent interlude with a handsome stranger at an unexpected time and place. You elaborate on the details.

- Your ideal lover, whether he is a real person or imagined, pursues you until you give in.

- You see a handsome man and seduce him. (Again, you fill in the details.)

Make a point of having these thoughts in "inappropriate" places—times and locations when sex would ordinarily be the last thing on your mind: at the supermarket, having dinner at mother's, while folding socks, and so on.

Use cues and props to help you out. Wherever you are, there is something in that room from which you can create a sexual image:

- A telephone: Someone calls you and suggests a drink, sex, a date. . .

- A doorknob: As it turns, imagine who is behind it and create a sexual encounter.

• A book: You open it and find a message inside from a secret admirer.

Be as romantic, as specific, or as lurid as you choose. Encourage whatever arouses you. Be as brief or as detailed as you wish.

Practice having erotic thoughts until it is easy to have at least one every hour. Enjoy them, and bask in the warm sensual feelings they evoke. (It's better than Valium.) Build sexual feelings back into your routine daily living so that they become a familiar part of your life.

Then, when he suggests sex, it won't be such a shock to your system. It won't jar your psyche. You may even start instigating some encounters yourself.

You may feel quite awkward at first. After all, any new skill you try for the first time—a foreign language, calculus, computers, whatever—is going to be awkward. Trying a new and erotic type of daydreaming can be as uncomfortable as the way you felt when you tried to order dinner in Spanish for the first time. The big difference is that with erotic fantasies you are actually relearning a long-forgotten pleasure.

If sexual fantasies hadn't been programmed out of you as a child, they would be there naturally. What can be programmed out can be programmed back in.

SPOTLIGHTING.   Another way to fill the fishbowl is with spotlighting. Spotlighting is a specific form of registering physical sensations and magnifying the effects. At any given moment your body is experiencing innumerable stimuli. However, you will only notice one or two things at a time.

Consider when you have a headache. If you get absorbed in something fascinating, and someone says to you, "How's your headache?" you have to think for a moment because you have momentarily forgotten it in your absorption with something else. That does not mean that the headache disappeared. It simply means that your focus of attention—your "spotlight"—was elsewhere, and you were not registering the uncomfortable feeling.

If you're sitting in a lecture hall listening to a speech, you probably won't hear the squeaky chairs and whispering in the background. If a siren goes by outside, you suddenly become conscious of traffic noise, and you'll start to tune out the lecture and may miss what's being said. So, no matter how interesting, pleasant, or exciting the experience you are involved in, when your mind shifts its attention even briefly to a new subject, the enjoyable sensations go out of focus.

You can tune out a headache and forget it's there until someone reminds you. You can sit in one position until your back aches or your buttocks hurt. Finally, the discomfort registers and you shift position. There are many other examples of the same reaction pattern.

We are so busy screening out sounds, noises, sensations, and emotions that the editing process has become well established. As a consequence, often when we want to feel, we can't. We think we feel everything that comes along, but often don't register many of the sensations that we are experiencing.

As a matter of fact, if people felt every single thing that was physically happening to them at any given moment, they would be driven to distraction in short order.

For normal day-to-day living, in fact for survival, one must screen out feelings. If you are constantly bombarded by all the feelings your body is experiencing at any given moment, you won't get much accomplished. However, in a sexual experience, editing (tuning out) feelings is undesirable. Thus, talent in one area becomes a handicap in another: a person who is excellent at editing out feelings (for example, someone who can suppress pain) is usually very poor at tuning specific feelings back in. Learning to counteract the tendency toward editing, through spotlighting, is essential to developing your sensuality.

To understand spotlighting, follow along with me for a few moments and attempt to focus your attention on the feelings I suggest. Sit down, and imagine your mind with a beacon attached to your forehead, like a miner's headlight. Anywhere you aim that light you become aware of the sensation in that area. Now, aim the imaginary spotlight back at your face and head. You'll feel the hair around your ears, the glasses on your nose, the collar around your neck. As you lower the spotlight, you'll feel the shirt on your back, the bra straps on your shoulders, the belt around your waist, the smoothness of the fabric that you are wearing. You'll feel, if you concentrate, pressure on your buttocks as you are sitting there. If you've been sitting for a long while, you might notice numbness or tingling.

Think for a moment about your feet. Can you feel your shoes? Of course you can. Were you thinking about your shoes five minutes ago? Does that mean they weren't there? Of course not. Spotlighting is required in order to capture feeling. You remember it through registering it. Conversely, we have a self-protective system to edit out or tune out feelings that are irrelevant to the moment.

During sex, spotlight on the physical feelings or you will miss them. Going through the motions or just being there is not enough.

If you think you're feeling everything that happens to you, try this test: Put your thumb and forefinger together. Use moderate pressure, not too light and not too hard. Don't rub them together. Just hold them steady. Close your eyes and spotlight on the feelings you are experiencing between the two fingertips. What sensations do you register? Nothing much? Is there warmth, pressure, firmness, smoothness? Some people can even feel their fingerprints. If you pay attention, you will feel a pulse. It didn't just arrive; it's been there all the time.

Open your eyes and think about how long it took from the time you first put your fingers together until you felt that pulse. Many things happen to us that we don't feel because we don't expect to feel anything, or because we're not paying attention.

Orgasms are like that. If you're not noticing the subtle, pleasurable feelings that are happening to you—that is, if you are not registering (spotlighting) them—they will not build into bigger feelings that may lead to the pleasure or an orgasm. Spotlighting is one of the most important techniques which can enable you to have orgasms.

Changing channels: Our fishbowl can only hold so much. What is most interesting is that it is never empty. It is like a vacuum where something floods in to fill the void. As a result, if the fishbowl is filled with distracting nonsexual or undesirable thoughts, the most effective way to get rid of them is to crowd them out with something else. In other words, consciously change channels. Draw on other thoughts. Fill the fishbowl by spotlighting physical feelings, or pleasant fantasy.

Active Touching

Just as spotlighting is one way of focusing on the physical sensations you are experiencing, active touching is another major way of enhancing your sensual experience. Active touching simply means to do the touching instead of being touched. With this technique you are not merely increasing your awareness, you are creating the sensual experience yourself. It is also a way to displace distractions from the fishbowl of your mind. If you are lying on your back being touched, it is far easier for your mind to wander than if your hands are active and you're concentrating on what you are doing.

The Art of Touching

Many women want to be touched and yet leave the pleasures of touching unexplored. They see touching as an effort, or as a "servicing" experience. That mind-set prevents them from discovering how directly enjoyable active participation in touching can be.

Touching is a form of nonverbal communication. It is a way of saying "I like you, I need you, I enjoy you, I love you, this feels wonderful."

The best approach to touching is to concentrate on pleasing yourself. Use some creative experimentation to make the touching more interesting for you. When the touching is planned solely to please the other person, it may not do so and often doesn't please the person doing the touching (you) either. Ironically, when you touch *for yourself,* you get much enjoyment from it and your partner usually enjoys it greatly, too. Not only will your touch please him, but he will derive pleasure from your enjoyment.

The scope of emotion that touching can express is far broader than words allow. Gentleness, tenderness, vulnerability, enthusiasm, vigorousness, excitement, passion are but a few of the feelings transmitted through touch. And don't forget that touching can be done with many parts of the body. Use your personal body language to communicate how you feel. Talk to him with your hands, your breasts, your lips.

Spectatoring

Sexual response is very sensitive to being watched. It can be easily inhibited, or significantly increased depending on the nature of the watching. Self-awareness can lead to self-consciousness if the view is a critical one.

THE NEGATIVE SPECTATOR. The fishbowl is often full of what is called negative spectatoring. Part of you is outside the experience looking in and judging what's happening. The monolog would go something like this: "He doesn't seem to be getting very erect. He could have spent a little more time doing that. I wonder what I'm doing wrong? I'm pretty dry myself. It doesn't look like I'm going to get very aroused. Wait a minute, some feelings are starting. Whoops, they disappeared. This is sure taking a long time. I wish he'd move his hand a little to the left and trim that hangnail. Well, it obviously isn't going to work. I just can't get going."

There you have the negative spectator: you giving yourself a running account of everything that's going wrong. That isn't very erotic.

THE POSITIVE SPECTATOR. You can improve matters by replacing the negative spectator with a positive spectator. Positive spectatoring is like looking in a mirror and watching yourself while you're having sex. That's a literal example. You can also do it with your mind.

Positive spectatoring is an attitude of silent approval. It is often erotic and will not detract from the sexual experience. For example, He: (thinking to himself) "Her skin feels so soft, it really turns me on." She: "I sure like the way he's touching me now. I enjoy it so much when these feelings start to build."

Devoted negators, however, will need a lot of practice to make the changeover: instead of criticizing everything with your mind, you must appreciate each detail—and savor every experience.

The fishbowl concept lets you substitute sexually fulfilling thoughts for sexually distracting ones. It's hard to think of *nothing* and, should you succeed, it dulls your sexual responsiveness. Crowd out those fears, that distress or that periodic anxiety, by focusing your conscious attention on images that will help to intensify your sexual experience.

THE TEN MOST COMMON REASONS WOMEN DO NOT HAVE ORGASMS (AND THEIR SOLUTIONS)

Reason	*Solution*
1. You try to hurry, thinking he's getting tired.	The harder you try, the more time it will take, so give in and enjoy yourself; and even if you don't have an orgasm every time, you'll have fun.
2. You expect a man to know what to do, and wait for it to happen.	Realize that he doesn't, and help him learn.
3. You don't know what you like.	Find out. Read books, talk to other women, and, most importantly, experiment with yourself.
4. You know what you want and won't tell him.	Tell him during sex; afterwards it's too late to do any good.
5. You lay there like Jell-O.	Make yourself move. Get on top. If you don't get physically involved, the odds are against having an orgasm.
6. You inhibit your reactions, afraid of rejection or embarrassment.	Give up trying to look beautiful. It's time to sweat and pant. Orgasms aren't elegant. Take a chance. Become vulnerable.
7. You try to please the man all the time.	Pay attention to pleasing yourself, too.

Reason	Solution
8. You endure discomfort or pain.	Don't assume pain or discomfort is normal, should be there, or isn't worth complaining about. Do whatever is necessary to get it fixed.
9. You are resentful and angry toward spouse.	If you can't solve your problems before sex, take an intermission from them during sex. You are only hurting yourself by holding onto the anger.
10. You are trying too hard.	When you try to make an orgasm happen, you don't allow it to happen. If you work at sex, it won't work. Make it fun again.

Roadblocks

There are many roadblocks to orgasm. Most of them can be removed by changing attitudes and behavior. However, it's useless to add a new technique or attitude without removing the old ones that have been getting in the way. Otherwise, it's like trying to go forward in a car with the brake on. Some of the questions and items in the following section are self-help checks intended to assist you in evaluating if some of the most common roadblocks exist for you.

Pain: if there is pain at any time, physiologically caused or due to the technique of your partner, you cannot expect to be orgasmic. If you're being polite, grinning and bearing discomfort while having sex, then you are also destined to remain unresponsive.

You can't expect to be aroused if it hurts, unless you happen to fall into a small segment of humanity with pathological sexual dysfunctions. If your partner is causing the pain or discomfort through too much pressure, or touching you in the wrong place—such as around the opening to the bladder—come to terms with your own sensations. Tell him.

Inertia: If you are not lubricating, you are not aroused. If you are not aroused, you are not going to reach orgasm. So ask yourself what you need to do to become aroused. If your body is passive and your mind and emotions are turned off, you cannot expect to respond.

Editing: If you're editing your responsiveness, as discussed above, you are unlikely to be orgasmic.

Pressure: If your mind is busy thinking of hurrying up, worrying that he is getting tired or bored, or if all your energy is being spent trying to wake him up and roll him over, your chances of reaching orgasm are nil.

Stop worrying about him and concentrate on yourself. If you're busy fretting that you're taking too long, that he may be bored or becoming emotionally disconnected from you, you're not likely to be very aroused. Shift your attention to your own feelings and tune out distractions—including him, if necessary.

In order to be orgasmic with a partner, you must:

1. Refuse to tolerate pain or discomfort.

2. Communicate your preferences in any way that works.

3. Take an active part in the experience.

4. Stop editing. Recognize when you are censoring out your full response—and counteract it.

5. Stop worrying about his feelings and sensations—and take an interest in yourself instead.

Short Cuts to Orgasm

Be your natural self—stop editing: You probably think, "I'm not editing," and you are probably wrong. What does editing mean? It means you are holding back in some way.

Remember the description of orgasm: the total body response. Consider how you react sexually when you're all alone, during self-stimulation. There is no one watching, no one to look good for, and no one to please—so you act naturally. You're paying attention to the feelings, enjoying them, and reacting however your body feels like responding. With your partner, whether you realize it or not, you are probably editing: not breathing quite so hard, trying not to sweat, smiling a little more to hide the wrinkles in your face. If the light is on, you're uneasy. You would like it dimmer—perhaps he's watching.

To have an orgasm, many body reactions need to take place and coordinate with one another. If you inhibit your body movement, resist breathing heavily, stretching, straining, panting, grunting, and groaning, chances are you won't have an orgasm either.

If you sincerely believe that you are not editing, there is a test you can do: masturbate in front of your partner. If you are able to be orgasmic alone when you masturbate, but not with him present, you are editing! If it takes longer with him, you are editing. Most women are very shy about this, and find it a difficult suggestion to follow. However, if you really want to be orgasmic with him, this is a short cut that will save you much therapy, money, time, and grief. This is a bridging step. Afterwards you'll be more easily orgasmic with him in other ways as well.

Have more sex—don't save yourself for later: The more sex you have, the more sex you will want, and the more sexually responsive you will be.

Contrary to popular belief in both men and women, the more you participate sexually, the more sexually interested and involved you remain and the more intense your sexual responsiveness becomes. It is a misconception that if you save your sexual feelings you'll have a more intense reaction the next time around. Not so. Similarly, women have been taught that if they masturbate they'll lose the ability to be orgasmic with intercourse, or that they may not have an orgasm at all the next time they're with a man. Nothing could be further from the truth. The more orgasms a woman has, the more she enjoys them regardless of the method. The more she "primes the pump," the more facile she becomes and the more interested in sex she remains.

Fail right: Your fears are probably the single most prominent reason you're not reaching an orgasm. You fear you won't have an orgasm. You fear he'll get tired, stop too soon, or come too fast. You fear that you will be rejected or thought abnormal. You fear you're not sexual enough to please him. You fear he'll lose his erection.

As Roosevelt and others have pointed out more elegantly, the only thing to fear is fear itself. If you allow the fear to take control of you, what you fear will probably come true. You *won't* be orgasmic. You *will* get tired. He *will* come before you do. You *will* have a self-fulfilling prophesy.

Once you identify the worst thing that could happen if you try (no orgasm, no arousal), you will realize that it is probably guaranteed to happen if you don't try. You have nothing to lose by getting involved. Anything that happens now is an improvement. So, let go of the fear, put it aside. You can't refuse to be fearful, but you can refuse to be preoccupied with the fear. You can say "Hello there, fear. I see you and I'm not going to let you govern my life." You thus set the fear in its place, recognize that it is there, and choose not to let it have the power over you that it has had until now. Sometimes just acknowledging the fear to your partner is a way to loosen its grip on you. "I'm afraid you will be angry if I don't come."

If you're going to fail, fail right. Throw yourself into the experience. Enjoy yourself. And if you're not orgasmic, you're not. But don't approach it by saying, "Gee, it isn't going to work anyway. There's no point in trying. I'm a failure." Because, in that case, you will be. Give it all you've got and take pride in the fact that if you fail you've done it right.

Say to yourself instead: "I'm not going to live tomorrow's problems today. If I reach orgasm, I'll be delighted. If I don't, it's no worse than what I have right now." Then, concentrate on the moment. It's terribly important to get rid of goals. If there is any goal, it shouldn't be the number of orgasms or the timing of orgasms, but to have a little fun. Set aside the goals and enjoy the journey. The odds for orgasm are much better. Remember, as long as you are enjoying yourself, you can't fail.

Lighten up: Don't be so heavy about sex. (I don't mean get up on your elbows.) It needn't be so serious. It's not a chore or an ordeal. Quit working at it so hard. Make it fun, and don't forget your sense of humor. Feel free to be playful too.

Prepare your body: See that you are physically comfortable during sex. If any position or activity is uncomfortable, stop the action immediately and make a change. If you're cold, cover up or close the window. If you're too dry, add a lubricant. If you're constipated, keep the thrusting rather shallow. In substance, cooperate with your body. Allow it to be at ease. Move with it, not against it. Don't be afraid of temporarily breaking the mood. Nothing can ruin a mood more effectively than a cold draft or a cramp in your leg. Fix the problem; the mood will return.

Be physically vigorous: Most women prefer the male astride position. It is relaxing. They can be lazy. It is not much work. However, most women reach orgasm more easily in the female astride position. There is a sound reason for this. When they are on top, their muscles are forced to participate: to contract and relax, to expend energy. *Body movement stimulates sexual reflexes.*

So be physically active. Give your body some energy and exercise. Get on top and use your muscles. Post! All of your body reactions respond more intensely and more rapidly if you have your muscles in gear. Sex is physical work. If you lay there like Jell-O, nothing will happen.

Learn to communicate: To communicate what you want, you must learn about yourself. Chapters 5 and 6 described how men and women can get to know themselves better emotionally. Many women are fairly ignorant about themselves sexually. Masturbation is a way of discovering and learning what you need from sex and how you feel about it—while you are in quiet comfort and solitude. There is nobody waiting for you, nobody watching you (except, perhaps, yourself), and no need for editing. Masturbating is part of taking responsibility for yourself, responsibility for becoming familiar with your own needs and your own responsiveness.

Take a risk: If you aren't sure what you would like, take a guess and then ask for it. For example: If you are having intercourse and nothing is happening, don't just lie there hoping he will figure something out. Choose another position, or ask him to stimulate your nipples. Your guess will be better than his. If you think of something you would like, try it. Don't say, "Oh, he wouldn't like it," or, "I guess I don't really need that; it's not so important." Chances are all those comments are just your way of avoiding the risk of embarrassing yourself. Take a chance!

Be resourceful: If things are not working out the way you expect, don't feel helpless. Use some imagination and ingenuity. A most impressive example of resourcefulness was demonstrated by John, who had been a paraplegic for five years. His wife left him two years after the accident. Determined to live and love, he forced himself to date, and eventually became quite a ladies' man. He was able to have intercourse even though he had no sensation below the waist.

One day he met a shy and reserved woman who was also paraplegic. He used his ingenuity and they managed to have intercourse in spite of all the obstacles, since neither could move their legs or hips. He had her lying on her back on a waterbed. He got on top in the "missionary position." He pushed down hard on his hands, which sent a wave down the bed, flipping her pelvis up and down. He wouldn't have found that method in any book.

In spite of the fact that neither of them could feel below the waist, being able to have intercourse together was good for their morale and provided an opportunity for intimacy and closeness.

Hand guiding: Once you have discovered what you like, there are many different methods of communicating your desires. Hand guiding is very important. It involves taking his hand in yours and showing him the pressure, the touch, the motion, and the specific area you prefer him to touch. It can be done by putting your hand on top of his, by placing your hand under his, or by intertwining your fingers so that while his hand is on top of or under yours, your fingers are side by side and you can grasp his hand with more control. It is like learning to dance together; a bit awkward at first, but if you practice and if you have patience, hand guiding becomes one of your most valuable and easy methods of transmitting information quietly and effectively at the moment that it's needed. Remember, also, that he can learn a great deal from watching how you touch yourself.

Talking: If guiding his hand doesn't do it, explain in words what you want and what you need: "I prefer this," or "a little to the left." Use your ability to express yourself to get your needs met. You must tell him at the time; mentioning it over a cigarette after sex won't do. You can't post-mortem an orgasm.

In communicating to your partner, the secret is to be direct, specific, and complete. Above all, show a little courage; take a few risks. Saying to a man, "Be gentle," is not enough. You have to show him what gentle means to you. What is gentle to him may be rough for you.

The World's Greatest Authority

A woman knows herself, how she feels, what she needs, what she fears, and what she enjoys far better than any outside person possibly could. By contrast to most other subjects in life, everyone is an authority on sex, sexual preferences, responses, and needs: their own.

You can express these needs verbally, by facial expression, with noises, or in many other ways—but especially through touching. No matter which way you choose to communicate those needs, it is absolutely essential to recognize that you are the world's authority on yourself, the president of your own "corporation." Others might make suggestions and offer educated guesses, and you may want to try them, but keep in mind that how you react to what they suggest will tell you in loud and clear tones whether or not their ideas are right for *you*.

Too many men and women, especially women, turn over responsibility for their behavior to someone else. It really can't be done, of course, but we let ourselves believe that it happens. "My psychiatrist says this is what I need. My sex therapist says I should have my legs together. My husband says I'm not like other women and I should be doing it this way. Harold Robbins says dig in your nails and draw blood. I don't do it that way— what's wrong with me?"

Those are all examples of abdicating your position as world's authority on yourself. What feels good to you, feels good to you. What feels bad to you, feels bad to you. You may not always know what you need, but if you look to yourself for the answers, the chances are good that you'll find them eventually.

Screen every piece of advice you read or hear from some other authority figure in the following manner: Does that fit me?

Is that how I have felt? What I would like? What I need? Does it make sense? Most important of all, ask yourself, "What have I got to lose by trying that suggestion?" If the answer is nothing, then try it. If, however, the answer is, "I could lose my life, my husband, it might cause me pain," etc., for heaven's sake don't do it based solely on trust. The "show me" philosophy is safe and sound.

Women have a terribly difficult time knowing what they want and need sexually because long, long ago they deferred the title of world's authority on themselves to the men of the world. Their reasoning was that "when the right man comes along, so will I." And they're still waiting. It's time to change the pattern.

What If He Won't Listen?

Now that you have become the world's greatest authority on your own sexuality, gotten rid of your fears, are your natural self, have lightened up, communicated, verbally and nonverbally—what if he still won't listen! What if his ego is hurt and he's ignoring your messages? It may seem to you he is acting this way, but you are probably misinterpreting him. In reality, your own fears may be getting in the way, but you blame him instead. Perhaps you find it awkward and uncomfortable to tell him or show him what you want, so you get out of it by saying he won't listen. If he isn't cooperating, the answer is to show him what you like as well as what bothers you. Men don't respond well to exclusively negative messages. For example, if you're going to say, "I don't like my breast touched like that," be sure to tell him how you do like it treated. "I like you to suck the nipple with your mouth while you massage my breast with your hand." Be specific. Be persistent. Don't assume if you tell him once he will remember forever. Keep in mind that he does not have the same sensations and anatomy that you do; and be fair, your needs may change from moment to moment. How is he to know if you don't tell him?

Don't make the mistake of thinking that he really *ought* to know, that if he weren't so retarded and clumsy you wouldn't have to go to all this trouble. He doesn't know. He probably isn't retarded or clumsy. A mind-set like that will only make you impatient, hurt his feelings, and quite possibly cause him to stop cooperating with you.

Everyone is looking for The Formula, the recipe for Success. Technique is important, but the skills that two caring people teach one another are far more important than some arbitrary, absolute series of steps from a distant authority. The guidelines in this chapter are meant to help teach you how to know yourself, discover your needs, ask for them to be met. Put them into practice for yourself, respecting your own uniqueness and enhancing your individual pleasure.

HOW NOT TO HAVE AN ORGASM

Relax your body and clear your mind.	(That way you'll be off in outer space, uninvolved and very bored.)
Don't tell him what you want.	(It takes longer when he has to figure it out himself—sometimes forever.)
Work at it.	(It will become such a chore you won't want to do it again.)
Lie there passively waiting for him to do it all.	(You may fall asleep.)
Endure pain.	(That will keep you awake.)
Don't tell him what you don't like.	(And then wonder why he's doing it.)
Think of your grocery list.	(Planning your dinner menus during sex will keep you occupied if he doesn't.)
Don't fantasize.	(You might think of someone else.)
Concentrate on pleasing him alone.	(And don't be surprised when he's the only one who's pleased.)
Only get involved if you feel romantic and in the mood.	(Otherwise you might end up having sex more frequently.)
Don't use artificial lubrication when you need it.	(If you use it, you will enjoy yourself so much you may start lubricating naturally.)

Don't masturbate.	(You might discover what you like before he does.)
Don't cheat. Follow somebody else's rules, not your own.	(Cheating doesn't exist except in your mind, or if you are engaged in some sexual Olympics and competing with someone else's idea of what sex should be.)
Don't sweat, grimace, grunt, or groan. But do fake orgasms.	(That tells him everything he's doing wrong is just right.)
Keep the lights out and don't look.	(That way you can pretend you are not really there, doing THAT.)
Inhibit your movements and act like a lady.	(You will be working harder and enjoying it less.)

A Section Especially For Men

Men have many questions about a woman's sexual reactions and needs. Some of them can only be answered by the woman herself, and men are encouraged to discuss these things with her.

What are the most sensitive areas of the woman's genitals?

Although women vary considerably, there are some generalizations that can be made: The clitoris and other external structures are usually the most sensitive. A test to do at home: Ask a woman friend, one who trusts you very much, if you can touch her on the inside of her thigh with the point of a pin. She will not feel pain, but will be aware of the pinprick sensation. It will feel the same on both thighs. As you bring the pin closer and closer to her genitals, the sensations will begin to be different. As the pin is touched to the labia majora, the hairy area of the lips of the vagina, the pinprick sensation will be slightly duller than it was on the inside of her thigh. If the pin is touched to the inside of the small lips, the labia minora, the vast majority of women will not feel the sharpness of the pin. Generally, they are absolutely astonished to find out that the sensation is dull.

The inside of the vagina is even less sensitive. It registers heat, warmth, stretch, and constriction but the ability of the vagina to perceive sensation is limited. In testing for that sensitivity from the outer thigh to the inner genitals there is a progressive decrease in feeling as you get closer to the vagina.

To make the situation both more complicated and less interesting, during the plateau phases of arousal there is a ballooning of the inner two-thirds of the vagina. Remember that the vagina actually becomes pear-shaped, with the inner section becoming slightly larger than the object (penis or whatever) contained inside. Consequently, neither the man nor the woman feels very much because the man is thrusting into a vacuum. The walls of the vagina do not touch the penis except at the entrance and perhaps the deepest part.

How important is penis size to a woman's satisfaction?

It is very important to some women, and not very important to others. Some women enjoy looking at and touching large penises. Most women, however, don't notice much difference during intercourse, although it matters to some. Women are considerably less concerned with penis size than are men, and the vagina is so flexible that it can accommodate a wide range of sizes. However, the larger the penis, the greater the chance of discomfort. In terms of ability to produce an orgasm, penis size makes little difference at all.

How do you find the clitoris?

The external genitals of the woman are small, vary in size, and are hard to see, especially in the dark. As a result, both men and women know very little about them. Everyone has seen diagrams of the area, usually in family life classes or school health programs. Although the sketches show the vagina as the outlet through which the baby comes, until recently there were no arrows on the drawings pointing to the clitoris. Many men and women still do not know where the clitoris is or what it looks like. A clitoris may look quite different from the drawings, or get lost in the folds of skin or hair. A foolproof way to find the clitoris is to locate the minor lips, which resemble petals surrounding the opening to the vagina. (These are small in some women, very large in others.) At the top of the lips, the two sides join in a V and blend right into the head of the clitoris. The top of each minor lip forks. One fork goes directly into the head of the clitoris and the other extends to form the hood covering the clitoris. Push the hood back slightly. Notice where the tips of the two minor lips meet at the head of the clitoris. You have now located the head of the clitoris.

How big is the clitoris?

The clitoris is about two centimeters or slightly longer. Most of it is located under the hood; only the clitoral head is easily seen. It is about the size of a small pea. A clitoris looks larger or smaller depending on how much is covered by the hood. If you feel with your finger from the exposed head and travel north, you will feel the rest of the clitoris under the skin. It resembles the texture of tendon.

Is it better for the woman if a man rides (thrusts) high?

It is not. Some men, in an effort to continue stimulating the clitoris during thrusting, attempt to thrust high. Unfortunately, all this does is crush the urethra—the opening to the bladder—which is located between the clitoris and the vaginal opening. It will frequently produce bladder infections (often referred to as "honeymoon cystitis") and kidney problems.

Do women prefer deep thrusting?

Not usually. Deep and vigorous thrusting is not necessarily the most enjoyable action for women due to the ballooning and the absence of significant sensation in the inner two-thirds of the vagina. (One patient refers to it as "incessant pounding.") It is the external pelvic bumping sensation produced by such enthusiastic thrusting that triggers some women to orgasm. Find out what *your* partner likes: ask her what feels good to *her*.

Why do some women not lubricate?

Lubrication has been a source of confusion and friction (in more than one sense). If a woman below the age of menopause does not lubricate, it is usually because she is not aroused. Some decrease in lubrication occurs after menopause, and sometimes requires supplementing with artificial lubrication. However, she is not likely to lubricate if she is thinking of other things—or if she happens to detest her husband at the moment. *It is normal not to lubricate if one is not aroused.*

However, she may actually be lubricating and not know it. Lubrication is produced inside the vagina, and some women lubricate quite copiously without realizing it. If they are lying on their back, the lubrication may form a pool in the back of their vagina, too far away to make insertion more comfortable and the sexual experience more pleasing. This situation can be resolved by dipping a finger into the vagina and drawing some of the lubrication out to coat the dry surface so that penetration is comfortable. The amount of lubrication varies from woman to woman. There is a wide range of normal. The fluid itself is clear and relatively odorless. Women's vaginal odors are due to their individual chemistry, sweat glands, time in cycle, the presence or absence of infections, and hygiene.

Some men, in an effort to determine if the woman is aroused, periodically stick a finger into the vagina of their partner to see if she is lubricating. This is not a very accurate method of determining how aroused she is, and is completely unnecessary unless you are both deaf-mutes. She is a person, not a car. A woman can usually tell whether you are "checking" or helping.

Why does the penis sometimes strike a "barrier" during intercourse?

The uterus itself moves up and down during the sexual response cycle. When it is down, the man's penis will bump into it. Some women enjoy having the penis thrust against their cervix. Others find it uncomfortable or painful. Do ask your partner how it feels to *her*. The bumping can either be a very pleasurable sensation or a deterrent to sexual arousal. If the impact against the cervix or uterus is painful, there is usually something wrong with the uterus. A low-grade infection or a minor problem may underlie the pain, so a medical examination is advisable.

Do women like a man to be rough with them, like biting their nipples?

For the record, and as a public service announcement, I ask the men of the world to please not bite nipples. Most women do *not* like to have their nipples nipped. It hurts. However, if you are a nipple biter and doubt my word, please ask her how she likes it. If she does, go right ahead. If she doesn't, believe her! (If you are his woman and say you like it when you don't . . .) It appears that every pornographic film has a hearty segment on nipple biting, with the woman clearly in throes of ecstasy over the event. Those are really throes of agony. Enough said.

Do It!

Reading this chapter will do you absolutely no good, if that is all you do. Put these recommendations into practice unless there is some harm in them for you or there are some serious objections from your partner. Ask yourself, "What have I got to lose by following these suggestions?" If the answer is, "Nothing but a little time," or, "I could embarrass myself," or, "I might feel awkward," remember that you have felt all of those things before and they're not so bad. So, do it and find out whether or not it works.

Men, give up the illusion that you have a "pipeline to God." Recognize that you can't do it for her or without her. Ask for her input, her help, and then listen to her. You can learn from each other.

The sexual techniques and approaches suggested may not make perfect sense to you, but try them anyway—at least once or twice—because that's the only way you'll find out if they are of any value.

Think about how you would advise a little boy who doesn't like carrots and won't eat them. He thinks carrots are yellow, ugly, and awful, but has never actually tasted one. One way to approach the problem is to encourage the child to make an educated choice. "Try one carrot and see. You might like the taste."

Children get irrational about carrots (and spinach). Adults get irrational about sex. Take yourself in hand, so to speak, and do something about it. Apply the same good reason and common sense to choices you make about sex as you do to other matters in your life. The effort will be worthwhile.

I can hear your excuses now. I've heard most of them before. "It's hopeless. His technique is so bad nothing will work . . ." "He doesn't turn me on . . ." "I'm just not in the mood . . ." "I have no interest . . ." "I don't feel like it . . ." "I'm angry with him all the time. As a matter of fact, I don't think I even like him . . ." "I certainly don't want to touch him . . ." "I see no point in masturbating, touching myself. That's not what I want anyway. I want a better sex life with him, not with myself . . ." "He has bad breath . . ." "I don't love him any more . . ." "It's too late . . ." "He won't cooperate . . ." "I'm tired . . ." "There's no time . . ." "The kids are awake during the day and at night I'm too tired . . ."

Men have an equally long list of excuses. "No matter what I do it won't help . . ." "I've tried that before . . ." "I can't last for two hours . . ." "Foreplay is boring . . ." "My other women didn't need that . . ." "It's her problem."

I could go on and on and on. Some of the excuses are valid, most of them are copouts. Even the "valid" excuses are essentially saying, "I'd really like to have an orgasm but it isn't high on my list. If someone gives me one as a gift, I'll take it, but I'd really rather not go to all the trouble and do the kinds of things necessary to bring it about myself."

If that is your choice, recognize it, assume responsibility for it, and don't make the effort. No one is forcing you. Not your husband, nor the sex experts of the world. It isn't necessary. You can and will live without it. However, if you would like to learn to become orgasmic, to have more orgasms, or to have them more quickly, it's time for you to quit thinking about it and start doing something about it.

Today, a woman who wants to fulfill both her biological sexual potential and the current sexual expectations of our society can have orgasms by self-stimulation, partner manipulation, or intercourse. It need not take her so long that either she or her partner gets tired. She will enjoy the total experience and usually reach her climax within ten to twenty minutes of erotic involvement. She will be able to have several orgasms in a row if she's in the mood to, or she can simply enjoy sex without any orgasms at all, if that is what she prefers at the time.

If it is within her repertoire to participate in oral sex, anal intercourse, and other variations on our usual themes, she also can learn to be orgasmic by those methods. Some women can become orgasmic within seconds through fantasy alone, or while doing something to their partner.

Bear in mind that while all of this is possible—if you want it—all of it is by no means necessary for a well-adjusted, even superlative sex life. People's standards and expectations are constantly changing, so instead of trying to keep up with every new idea, find out what pleases you the most and enjoy it.

CHAPTER 12

The Impotence Epidemic, Premature Ejaculation, and Ejaculatory Incompetence
His problem, her distress

Impotence isn't contagious, rarely fatal, but can be life-threatening. It affects men at any age and devastates them. Because of impotence, a man can become depressed, and sometimes even suicidal.

Premature ejaculation is a common occurrence and is now considered one of the most easily treated sexual problems. Impotence, depending on the cause, is a close second. Ejaculatory incompetence is less common and more difficult to correct. Even though it is hard to talk about one without including the other, they are not variations of the same theme. They are distinctly different problems, but because they are controlled by the autonomic (automatic) nervous system, understanding this neurological system is helpful in treating the problems sensibly.

The Automatic Nervous System

You have two nervous systems. One is under voluntary control. That's the one that says, "move, arm," or "close, eyes," or "walk," and your arm moves, your eyes close, you walk. You have very good control over that. Alcohol interferes with this system, and police prove it by having you attempt to walk a straight line.

The other system is involuntary (automatic). It is in charge of running your body, whether you are paying attention or not. It makes you breathe whether you are thinking about it or not. It controls your heart rate, the size of your pupils, blood flow to the intestinal tract, blood flow to the skin and other organs. Most of us have very little control over this nervous system.

The autonomic system is divided into two portions—the *sympathetic* and the *parasympathetic*. These two systems do opposite things to your body. The sympathetic system is very easy to remember because it is in charge when you need action: the flight, fight, and fear response. The parasympathetic system is in charge when your body is calm.

In order to understand the sexual mechanism, let us explore how each system affects different parts of the body, particularly sex.

THE SYMPATHETIC SYSTEM.   When trying to understand the sympathetic nervous system, think of the survival reflex: flight, fight, fear. What do you think the sympathetic nervous system does to pupil size? It would dilate them. You need to be able to see danger better if you're going to escape or fight, so your peripheral vision is increased. What would happen to blood flow to the skin with increased sympathetic activity? It decreases, because the last thing you need is blood flow to your skin if you're going to fight—you would bleed more. If you're going to flee, you need that blood in your leg muscles instead. What about the digestive system? It shuts down. If you're fighting flighting, or fearing, the last thing you need to do is digest food.

So, your sympathetic system causes your pupils to dilate so that you can see danger coming, and your heart to beat faster in order to circulate blood to essential organs. Your circulation shifts, letting the blood vessels in your skin constrict. That is why when you are afraid, you become pale, cold, and clammy. The blood is shunted away from skin structures—to the deep muscles for running, to the lungs for oxygenation, to the heart for pumping. Less blood is allotted to the brain, the digestive tract, or any other structures not essential at that moment. Face it, in a survival situation, how necessary is your penis?

For the purpose of this discussion, your cardiovascular system considers your penis a superficial skin structure. The vessels respond to the sympathetic system and constrict. The erection is lost almost immediately.

THE PARASYMPATHETIC SYSTEM. The sedentary activities such as digestion, and erection, are, by and large, parasympathetic activities.

Ejaculation is under the control of the sympathetic system. While it may not be intuitively obvious at first, it is very sensible once you think about it. Imagine yourself as a caveman two million years ago, out in the glade fornicating with a cavewoman. A saber-toothed tiger leaps out of the foliage. Your sympathetic system signals danger and adrenalin surges through your system. It says: "Ejaculate and run for the hills," or "Lose your erection, leave the woman behind and head for safety."

The "adrenalin reflex" has just taken effect.

The Adrenalin Reflex

Loss of erection is not an indication of a failure of masculinity, and should not cause self-condemnation. Rather, new and previously unpublished research indicates that it has valid psychophysiological roots.

Loss of erection actually results from a chemical within our body triggered by fear. An emotion (fear) causes a chemical (adrenalin) to instantly appear in your bloodstream. *Our mind causes chemical and physical reactions in our body.* This is not just theory, it is fact! It is well known that stress contributes to ulcers, heart disease, and impotence—each of which in turn increases the stress on the body system.

Until recently, the mechanism involved in impotence, not caused by trauma or disease, has not been well understood. The adrenalin reflex, however, explains it in a clear and sensible fashion.

Most people know that when they are suddenly frightened, when they have been almost run over by a car, adrenalin—the survival chemical—instantly surges through their system, preparing the person for "fight or flight." Adrenalin results from an emotion and appears instantly in the bloodstream.

Adrenalin causes specific physical reactions within the body. It causes impotence by directly constricting the blood vessels in your penis—just as it does those in your skin—and the erection is lost. The more upset you get about it, the more adrenalin pumps into your system, and the more impossible it is to become erect again.

Another effect of adrenalin on sex is to stimulate ejaculation. That is why an anxious man will ejaculate faster than one who is at ease. Extreme fear can cause ejaculation. Men who are about to be executed have ejaculated—hardly an erotic experience. Some men report ejaculating during physical exertion, such as a man who said: "When I was sixteen I was climbing a rope, trying to beat everybody else, and I ended up ejaculating instead."

I was taking a calculus exam, and during the exam, I ejaculated two times. What is wrong?

A very strong sympathetic response, due to fear or stress, can cause ejaculation when there is not even erotic feeling. Such men are anything but aroused at the time.

Performance Anxiety

A major cause of psychological impotence is fear of performance. A man who is worried whether or not he is going to get erect, or whether he will measure up to other men, or whether or not he will be able to make his partner orgasmic is pumping adrenalin into his system. The chemical prevents him from getting erect in the first place (or causes him to lose his erection shortly after penetration). The more upset he gets that the erection isn't there, the more impossible it becomes for him to become erect at all. He discovers that he cannot will an erection, and begins to suspect that something is physically wrong with him. He may have no use for psychologists, and doesn't believe that it is all in his mind.

It isn't.

By the time he loses the erection, the inhibiting chemical process has already taken place. Stress, anxiety, or fear releasing adrenalin into the bloodstream constricts the vessels in the penis and causes loss of erection. Anxiety triggers the adrenalin reflex into motion.

CASE HISTORIES: A couple has been married approximately twelve years, and the wife has never been orgasmic with intercourse. He is a rapid ejaculator. For years he works to make her orgasmic. His concern grows as time passes. He wonders if it is him or her. The more stress that develops, the faster he ejaculates. Stress also increases the chance that he will become impotent, because he is no longer enjoying himself. Each situation represents psychological failure.

As anxiety increases, the human male finds that the erection begins to occur a bit more slowly, until, one evening he does not get an erection at all. It can happen to the eighteen-year-old boy on his first sexual encounter: he is with a girl he wants to impress. He's worried, concerned, and fearful because he doesn't know what to do—therefore, no erection.

A twenty-year-old who has functioned fine since he was sixteen becomes impotent with a prostitute. His religious or ethical background makes him unable to respond. He feels stress and anxiety—therefore, no erection.

Somewhere along the line, failure to achieve or maintain an erection occurs. And thus begins the *fear of future failure*. Such fears are irrational, but real. A man hits twenty home runs in a row, then strikes out once. His next turn at bat he is not thinking: "Will I hit a home run?" He is worrying: "Will I strike out again?" He reacts the same way with sex: after one failure he says, "My God, I'm impotent." If he was treating sex as a natural function, he would not become impotent. If he is unable to urinate in a crowded men's room, he doesn't say, "My God, I'll never urinate again." He understands the pressures of that circumstance and knows that he will function normally next time.

Instead, to make sure that he is successful in his next sexual encounter, he fortifies his courage with a few drinks of alcohol, which almost guarantees that he will not respond.

After a few failures, the next stage may be to avoid the issue altogether, by rarely entering into sexual activity unless his wife or girlfriend presses him. Sometimes he does a test run himself—only to find his penis won't cooperate. He has developed a rampant case of performance anxiety.

Why is it that during foreplay I have a good erection, and lose it when it really counts? What is wrong?

Picture the toreador, with his cape, making his passes, and then when he takes the sword out, at the moment of truth . . . that is the moment of fear. That's the moment of performance pressure, and that's where failure most commonly occurs: either at the moment of penetration, a moment before, or right afterward—whenever your adrenalin reflex occurs.

How many men are impotent?

It's difficult to find reliable data. A conservative estimate is 10,000,000 men in the United States. It is probably much higher.

Does age cause impotence?

No. As a man passes forty the chances of illness and disease increase with each decade. The main reason that age effects the percentage is medical. A man who retains a good state of mental and physical health can look forward to enjoying sex throughout his lifetime.

Alcohol and Sex

Alcoholism is still a disease that is very poorly understood and it is classified in many different ways. One of these is the alpha-beta-gamma-delta scale. The alpha alcoholic is one who gets into trouble from alcohol: gets drunk driving tickets but still functions well. At the delta end of the scale you have the skid-row drunk, with the big liver and the yellow eyes. Alcohol does affect the ability to be erect, but how it affects a given individual depends on where that person is on the scale. A light drinker may be helped by alcohol. If a drink or two relieves anxiety (short-circuits the adrenalin reflex), it may enable him to become erect more easily. However, it is generally not a very good idea to try for "Dutch courage," since, in fact, alcohol actually decreases the ability to be erect. To quote what Shakespeare said in the 1500s, alcohol provokes desire, but takes away the performance. Experiments have confirmed his wisdom whether we're talking about rats, mice, dogs, or humans.

Even a very few drinks can interfere with the ability to get erect. It is one of the most common causes of impotence. The more years of drinking the greater the chances for physiological impotence.

If you are a heavy drinker, all the psychotherapy in the world won't help your erections unless you stop drinking.

Another Self-Fulfilling Prophesy

Think about how we trap ourselves. Consider someone preparing for an important examination: a bar exam, the real estate licensing test, medical school finals. Fear of failure is so great that the student says, "Well, I'm not going to pass anyway." The person procrastinates (just as the impotent man avoids sex), finally getting so anxious that any attempt to read or study is useless. The individual can't absorb what his eyes are seeing. The odds are pretty slim that a student who handles fears in this fashion is going to pass. Men do the same thing in trying to have an erection. They say, "I'm going to fail so there's no point in trying."

On the other hand, if the same student says, "Well, yes, I'm afraid that I might fail, but if so, I'm going to fail right! I will study as much as I can, give it my full attention, and use all the hours before the exam in my best effort. I'm not going to worry about failing because all that will do is help it happen. I'll face the fact if I have to. In the meantime, I'm going to concentrate on the present, and study hard." That student has a chance. If the impotent man assumes that attitude, so does he.

The Spectator

Closely associated with fears of performance is the negative spectator discussed in Chapter 11. With sex, as we have said, everybody is a spectator to some degree.

The positive spectator enjoys watching his partner or himself during sex. That's why some people put mirrors on their walls or ceilings. They enjoy watching themselves. Many people feel guilty about that, as though it were some sort of unhealthy, voyeuristic activity, but it's not. A certain amount of lighting can bring out the positive spectator in most individuals and make that sexual experience much more stimulating.

The negative spectator is the individual watching his or her own "performance." This man is in bed with himself, gauging, judging, and watching. He asks himself, "Will I get an erection? If I get it, will I keep it? If I keep it will I keep it long enough?"

Sex Must Be Sexual

Sexual feelings have to be there in order for the automatic sexual reflexes to begin.

People often forget that sex, by its very nature, has to be sexual. It must be erotic. The concept is so simple that we ignore it; yet it is essential to satisfying sex.

Conversely, any input that is nonerotic, nonstimulating, is nonsexual. Fear, negative spectatoring, performance anxieties, work, and obligations are not erotic to most people and will inhibit arousal. The more these concerns for performance and concerns for failure filter into the brain, the less ability the person has to be erect.

For some, love is unfortunately part of the list above, as in the Madonna syndrome. Some people's problems are due to the fact that the acts and images that are erotic to them are not compatible with their notion of love.

What is the relationship between extramarital intercourse or a prostitute experience and impotence?

Many men will go outside of a relationship for the first time to check themselves out. They have had a failure and want to find out who is responsible: they are asking, "Is it me, or am I not finding her as sexually attractive as I once did?" About 80 percent of the time, the answer is, "yes it is me." The other 20 percent of the time the male is able to function, because he doesn't care about the woman and is not anxious to please her. In other words, he is not performing for anybody. He is doing it for himself for a change. The terrible irony is that, rather than recognize that he was able to function beautifully in an extramarital relationship only because his emotions were not involved and he was having fun, he blames his wife: "It is her fault our sexual relationship has deteriorated. She doesn't appeal to me."

Using the fishbowl concept described in Chapter 11, let's examine the brain of a male who is becoming aroused. A voluptuous female is in view. Her image causes his brain to generate erotic thoughts. He absorbs the stimulating mental picture; then he adds to it memories and images from his own store of erotic experiences. Next, he puts in whatever anticipations he might have and the mixture becomes even more erotic. Eventually his brain is almost full of sexual thoughts. As it continues to fill—he is now not only with her, but he is holding hands, kissing—he is becoming more and more interested and excited. This man will get erect. When his brain fills with erotic thoughts, he becomes naturally aroused.

Now, let's explore the mind of a man who has had one, two, forty, or even two hundred failures to be erect. The same process occurs in his mind, but as he gets closer to having intercourse, he starts to worry: "Oh-oh, I'm getting turned on. I'd really like to have sex, but will I be able to perform?" Performance anxiety turns on the negative spectator instead of his penis. When less than half of his brain is occupied with the anticipation of pleasure, it is no surprise to find that he is either only half erect, or not erect at all.

The Woman's Reaction

When a man becomes impotent the woman reacts in predictable ways. After a while his anxiety unleashes a negative spectator in her. She begins to worry about his erection too. Eventually the anticipation of walking into the bedroom and enjoying herself, of holding close, of intercourse, transforms into fear of failure. Negative anticipation finally develops avoidance patterns in both of them.

She may take longer to become aroused or not even become sexually involved for fear that she will just become frustrated: "He's not going to get an erection and I'll be left hanging." So she becomes a negative spectator and takes longer to become aroused.

She watches him berate himself, because that is usually what he does. She doesn't say he is inadequate, he says it to himself (and to her)—probably because he wants to criticize himself before she gets a chance. He kicks himself around the bedroom and tears his hair, apologizing for being a failure—he is tortured and miserable. She is more bothered by his reaction than his impotence. The situation becomes less and less erotic for her, and she begins to avoid him. Pretty soon both of them develop sexual aversion.

The woman invariably blames herself. Is he impotent because of me? Her self-image is shaken: "Doesn't he find me sexually alluring? Am I getting old? Am I no longer attractive to him?" And the older she is, the more concerns she has about her own body. She may have gained ten or fifteen pounds in the last twenty years, is not quite as voluptuous as she once was, has some skin folds, or a few stretch marks from delivering children. He tries to tell her how lovely she is, but she doesn't believe him. No matter what he says, it doesn't reassure her. She either avoids sexual activity with him or has an extramarital affair to prove that she is still sexually desirable to someone.

Someone once told me that the woman controls the man's erection. Does the woman's technique or the man's psyche determine whether he reaches total erection?

Nobody can control anybody else's natural function. Saying that I control a male's erection would be like saying to someone, "I make you hungry," or "I make you thirsty." Reactions are determined by whatever that individual takes in, not by the stimulus alone. If I serve liver and onions to a group of people, half of them would love it and the other half would hate it. It's because of the way they perceive it, not because of what I put out here. A woman may serve a good meal, but she doesn't control the man's erection unless his mind is receptive. The best technique won't work if he is preoccupied by his fears, and trapped in the adrenalin reflex.

Elephants

If I said to you right now, "Don't think of elephants," wouldn't you immediately have elephants on your mind? Herds! However, if I said, "Don't think of elephants," and proceeded to tell you an incredibly fascinating story about giraffes, time would pass rapidly without any elephants on your mind (maybe a straggler or two).

The impotent man must learn how to tell himself a fascinating sexual story, and get rid of his elephants (fears). Telling him what to avoid is not enough: saying "Don't be frightened, don't worry about performance, don't be a negative spectator" is like saying "Don't think of elephants."

Fill that fishbowl with erotic thoughts instead.

Fantasy: Antidotes to Elephants

Some men enjoy fantasy. Others think it is only necessary if something has gone wrong with their wife—she's too fat or too old. Fantasy can be many things. You are sitting on a couch with a woman, petting and getting aroused. You take her hand and lead her to the bedroom. What is going on at that moment in both your minds is fantasy—the fantasy of what each of you expects to occur in the next five or ten minutes.

Anticipation is a type of fantasy. Looking forward to pleasure is a fantasy, whether you visualize it with the person that you're with, or fantasize something that you would like to be doing with someone else.

Fantasy is a tool used frequently in therapy to help men rid themselves of performance anxiety, fear of failure, and negative spectatoring. Erotic thought substitution (fantasy) is an excellent antidote to elephants.

Impotence: Is It Physical or Psychological?

Psychological impotence is based on the fact that a man's sympathetic system is acting up. Because he is stressed or fearful, he is not able to use his mind in a way that is sexually effective. Most men who come to see me for impotence hope that it is a physical problem. They want some pill, shot, or medicine to cure them. They don't realize that of the two forms of impotence, the physical type is usually by far the most serious. There are many causes of organic (physical) impotence: diseases, drugs, physical injury. And, to make matters worse, if a man is organically impotent for *any reason*, he also becomes psychologically impotent. He doesn't know it is medical at first, and so he inherits all of the fears of performance, fears of failure, and negative spectatoring.

Sometimes It Isn't What It Appears to Be

Several years ago, during a lecture to a group of lawyers, I mentioned that diabetes can lead to organic impotence. In fact, the incidence of impotence is about five times higher in diabetics than nondiabetics. That night, a thirty-four-year-old attorney with diabetes, who had never had any sexual difficulty before, became *psychogenically* impotent. The power of suggestion is incredibly strong, especially when a man already has a physical susceptibility. Six months later, this man finally came to see me. It was clear that he had started down the road to nonfunctioning many years earlier. A slight psychological nudge was all that was needed for him to quit functioning altogether. In this case, his sexual interaction with his wife had been stressful for years, and the information that diabetes could cause impotence triggered a self-fulfilling prophesy.

Fortunately, when there is no physiological disorder and the problem hasn't been there too long, it can be cured in a short time. In this case, the man was functioning normally again within a few weeks.

Widower's Syndrome: Use It or Lose It

This form of impotence occurs to a man who has lost his wife through a lengthy wasting-away disease. Sexual functioning goes relatively well as long as he is able to have intercourse with his wife. If, however, during the last two to three years of the marriage, his wife is too ill to participate in intercourse, the syndrome begins.

Out of deference to her, he doesn't approach her sexually. He doesn't masturbate because that has never been his pattern. And, he loves her too much to even consider an outside affair.

Following her death, and a mourning period, he begins to date again. When the first opportunity to have intercourse with a lovely, energetic widow comes along, he finds he is impotent and completely unable to function. He is absolutely astounded. This man has never had a day of sexual difficulty in his entire life. He may be in his late fifties, early sixties, even in his seventies or eighties, but he has never thought of himself as old. Now, he begins to wonder if he's over the hill and just didn't know it until now. Age alone, however, is not a barrier to sexual enjoyment: the oldest man studied in the Masters and Johnson laboratory was ninety-two; he had intercourse several times a week and masturbated in addition to that.

If a man in his fifties or sixties for whatever reason puts his sexual functioning on the shelf, he is asking for problems. If he does not masturbate or have intercourse, he eventually faces a "use it or lose it" phenomenon. Put another way, if you place an arm in a cast for six weeks—even if there was nothing at all wrong with it—you will not be able to pitch nine innings of baseball on the day the cast is removed. Our bodies simply don't work that way.

Our widower, who has put his sex life on the shelf for three years, changes his mind one day, and expects everything to work. Biology doesn't cooperate. The surprise is that he is surprised. He wouldn't be if he treated sex like other natural functions. Widower's syndrome can be cured in most cases, but the longer a man has gone without functioning the more difficult he is to treat.

As a man ages, unless disease intervenes, or interest disappears, he can expect to continue to function well sexually. There are some specific changes that he can expect, but none interferes with the ability to enjoy intercourse. The full erection is not as firm as when he was a young man (for example, a grade 10 at eighty or ninety would be more like a grade 8 at twenty). The volume of the ejaculate and the force of the ejaculate decrease; the urge to ejaculate each time is not so strong. A seventy-year-old might still enjoy intercourse two or three times a week, but wish to ejaculate only once. Also, the refractory period increases. A man who could ejaculate within an hour of his last orgasm as a youth may have a refractory period of many hours, or a day, when he is in his seventies. The quantity of sex may decrease slightly with age, but many older men say the quality increases.

Healthy seventy-year-olds have intercourse approximately twice a week, and thirty-year-olds average about once a week. Shocking, isn't it? The reason is that thirty-year-olds are out there slaying dragons, making a living, being angry at their wives or husbands, and having all the other difficulties and joys of living together and raising children. At seventy, there is time for each other, and—assuming both are healthy—an opportunity to enjoy sex.

Let Your Fingers Do the Walking

If a man does not masturbate, he is encouraged to begin. Self-diagnosis is much more difficult otherwise. Usually, I will suggest that he masturbate two to four times a week, in order to find out how he functions sexually by himself.

The least threatening sexual situation is usually when an individual is alone. You are not performing for anybody else, so the fears of performance are minimized. You haven't removed them yet, however, and some difficulty may exist.

But what if you don't masturbate? The sensation in the genitals is different under different circumstances. During a morning shower, your genitals feel different from when you are erotically involved. Some men have never masturbated. Many males have to relearn how to masturbate, because they have not done it for so many years or because they negatively spectate with masturbation just as successfully as they negatively spectate with intercourse.

Once you have mastered solitary masturbation, mutual masturbation is the next step. If you're just playing and touching, but not planning on going on to coitus, there is less pressure than with intercourse and you may function better. Many men and women have never tried it. Has your husband ever been ejaculated by your hand? Has your wife ever ejaculated you by hand?

The Etiquette of Ejaculation

Both men and women often have negative feelings about the semen itself. Because men grow up hiding their ejaculate, fearing that they're going to be caught masturbating, they sometimes get married with the attitude that they should conceal it from their wife too. If they ejaculate accidentally, they'll jump out of bed, grab some toilet tissue, and wipe it up.

Women get the idea that something is wrong, too. It becomes

an embarrassment and makes intercourse the only "right" way to interact. When intercourse is the only alternative, it excludes a multiplicity of activities, such as masturbation, mutual masturbation, genital-oral sex, anal intercourse, etc. With genital-oral sex, a man is not as worried about pleasing his partner. If he is able to enjoy it, he is not at the moment concerned about her orgasms or his erection, because it is for his pleasure even if she is enjoying doing it. So many men who have difficulty being erect with intercourse due to performance pressures, are able to be erect with oral sex because they're able to lie back and relax and not worry about their erections. On the other hand, some are unable to be erect at all because they are feeling worked upon and are nervous being "done to."

The Peter Meter

One of the newest diagnostic methods for determining whether the cause of impotence is psychological or physiological is the Nocturnal Penile Tumescence (NPT) monitor, more fondly referred to as the Peter Meter. It is a portable machine that a patient takes home with him at night to measure the number of erections he experiences during sleep. As described in Chapter 2, the average healthy man should be erect approximately 20 percent of sleep time. If this test shows no erections at all, the man probably has a physical problem. Although the NPT monitor does not indicate whether the problem is caused by nerve damage, hormone deficiencies, drugs, etc., it will show that something physical is involved. If the test is normal, the erection problem is probably mental (the adrenalin reflex).

My doctor told me I needed testosterone shots, but they didn't work. Why?

Let us assume that a patient has a physical problem due to a testosterone deficiency. His NPT monitoring is flat. Testosterone injections are begun, but there is no physical improvement. As mentioned earlier, testosterone takes a few weeks to do its work. But months pass, and there is still no improvement. What could be wrong in the treatment of this patient? Think back to the adrenalin reflex. If a man is still stressed because he is worried that the treatment won't work, or simply anxious because it hasn't worked yet, the adrenalin reflex will ensure that he won't become erect no matter how much testosterone he is given.

On the other hand, let us assume that testosterone is given to a patient who is psychologically impotent and doesn't actually require any testosterone. This patient believes the shot will help him, and becomes potent again overnight. The testosterone has "treated" the adrenalin effect successfully. However, a water shot would have done just as well (if the man truly believed it would help) and would have been less risky.

One can usually distinguish the difference between organic impotence and psychogenic impotence by measuring nocturnal penile tumescence.

The NPT monitor produces a strip of paper just like an EKG—but instead of heart tracings, the tracings show the degree, quality, and duration of erections. There are many criteria for reading these strips, but in general the study determines if erections are present, and contributes valuable information to the diagnostic workup.

If there is no nocturnal penile tumescence, or if it is less than the normal amount for your age group, the erection problem is probably physical rather than psychological. If the NPT tracing is normal, you are wired together correctly and the problem is probably psychological. However, a thorough physical examination and laboratory procedures including studies of hormones (including testosterone) and tests for diabetes should also be done.

The Poor Man's NPT

A less precise home study can be done for just a few cents. Before bedtime, take a roll of stamps and bend them several times at the perforations. Then moisten them and stick them around the base of your penis with one overlapping stamp. If, when you wake up in the morning, the stamps are broken, you have evidence of some erections.

Diagnostic Errors: Man Vs. Machine

As an example, the NPT strip on a thirty-two-year-old male who had been impotent for three years showed a normal tracing. He had multiple sclerosis and on the basis of his neurological disease had been diagnosed as being organically impotent.

NPT monitoring showed this conclusion to be incorrect. During the test, he spent 25 percent of the night completely erect. (See Figure 1.)

Yet when I had asked that male if he ever woke up with morning erections, he answered no, because he doesn't happen to have an erection just before he awakens. The completely flat baseline shows the point when this man woke up. (See Figure 2.)

Many men who don't think they get nighttime erections demonstrate by NPT that they actually do.

A twenty-eight-year-old male came to see me with diabetes mellitus. Because he had only had the disease for two years, was relatively young, and was under good control with medication, he had been diagnosed as having a psychological disorder.

A physical examination, however, revealed a different picture. The diabetes had caused many complications, resulting in nerve loss in his extremities, including his penis. A penile tumescence study on this individual confirmed the problem as physical. It showed eight hours of flat line—no erections at all. (See Figure 3 for excerpt of this tracing.)

But Please Don't Overlook the Medical

This man was organically impotent, and no amount of psychotherapy in the world is ever going to correct it. I can't overemphasize how important it is to make a correct diagnosis in order to recommend the right therapy. Without the proper diagnosis, this diabetic man might have gone through years of unnecessary psychoanalysis, wasted time and money, and developed psychic anguish because he wasn't getting better in treatment.

Treatment

The psychological therapy for impotence is almost identical to the treatment of difficulty with orgasm in the woman. If you review that chapter and just reverse the sexes, the same techniques will work for you.

Pressure, negative spectatoring, and working at sex are the

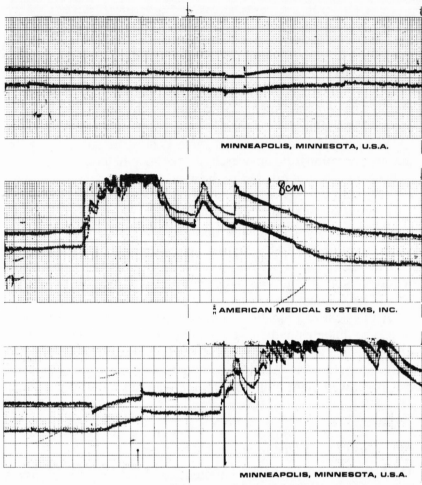

MINNEAPOLIS, MINNESOTA, U.S.A.

8cm

ᵃⁿ AMERICAN MEDICAL SYSTEMS, INC.

MINNEAPOLIS, MINNESOTA, U.S.A.

FIGURE 1. Excerpt from NPT tracing of psychologically impotent male

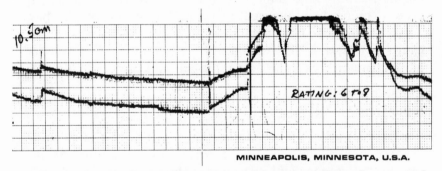

10.5cm

RATING: 6 TO 9

MINNEAPOLIS, MINNESOTA, U.S.A.

FIGURE 2. Excerpt from NPT tracing of impotent patient who reported the absence of nighttime erections and morning erections

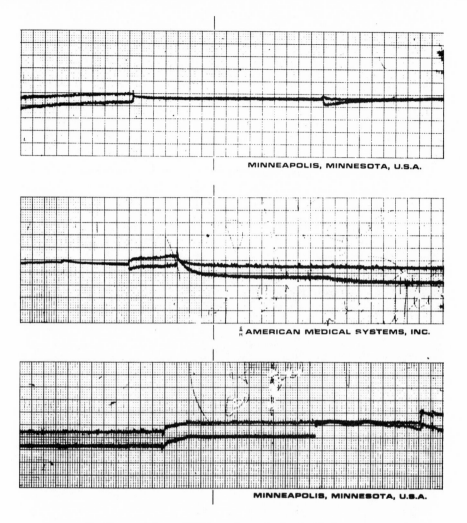

FIGURE 3. Excerpt from NPT tracing of physically impotent male

worst offenders. The antidotes are tuning in, positive spectatoring, focusing, fantasy, and most important, comfort. If you don't recognize the physical and emotional conditions you require for comfort, you cannot meet those needs. Reflect and consider until you search them out. Then put them into action.

Remember that if you are chronically depressed, fatigued, worried, or angry, these feelings will probably sabotage your erections until you resolve them.

The definition of impotence is "failure 50 percent of the time." That doesn't mean you should wait until you are at that level to do something about it—any more than you would wait until you had pneumonia to treat a cough.

Most men get pretty unhappy if they lose even one erection, or can't respond when they have the desire and the opportunity.

Have a Conversation with Your Penis

Impotence is your penis talking to you. Listen to what it is telling you. If it is not erect when you think it should be, if it won't ejaculate when you want it to, any one of several things could be going on.

- You are not aroused.
- You are anxious.
- You are fatigued.
- Too much alcohol.
- Drugs—legal or illegal.
- You are depressed.
- You don't find her emotionally or physically appealing, and neither does your penis.
- You are angry or resentful with her; your penis is pouting.
- You are expecting it to perform under hostile circumstances.
- Your penis is not a trained animal act; it will not jump when you say so.
- You are sexually aversive.
- You are physically uncomfortable.
- There is something medically wrong.

A headache tells you: "Slow down, stop reading, rest your eyes, take some aspirin, don't drink so much tonight, and if the pain doesn't go away, see a doctor. Maybe something else is wrong."

Your limp penis sends you a similar message: "You are getting unhappy, you drink too much, you are disregarding your feelings, you are trying to prove something rather than experience it, you are working at sex, you are more preoccupied with her reaction than your own (and you are probably getting neither)."

If you listen—especially to the earliest cues—you can respond to the situation and keep it from progressing.

Dr. Bernie Zilbergeld in his book, *Male Sexuality*, suggests that your penis write you a letter. Try to see the world from its point of view for a few moments. The letter might go something like this:

> Yes! I have a few complaints. It's about time you asked! I have been trying to get your attention for years. Now I can't even look you in the eye anymore. That beer belly has to go. I am so ashamed of how you look, I don't want to be seen with you. Besides, after all you drink to get your courage up, I get so dizzy, I can't walk, much less stand up straight. And about your taste in women, after a few belts you must go blind. I am not about to associate with the types you choose.
>
> Then you go home to your wife and breathe on her. Is that in hopes that she will fall down before you do? No wonder she runs you off. You say it's her fault: You wouldn't drink so much if she gave you more sex. Well, you *know* she won't let you near her when you have been drinking, so you have a convenient way to blame her both ways: if it weren't for no sex you wouldn't drink, and since you drink, there is no sex. Convenient for you, isn't it? As a matter of fact, until you clean up your act, I am retiring. Don't count on me to keep you company. Straighten up, and so will I!

Impotence eventually becomes a habit. Adaptations and adjustments are made. Rationalizations help maintain the status quo. Blaming someone else justifies another drink, a few more hours at work, or an affair.

It is difficult for most men to go in for help. But, fellas, if you haven't been able to help yourself, and it has been a few years, it's time!

You may have to sort through a few professionals until you find one who will do. A quick trip to the urologist, or sending your wife in to get "fixed," usually doesn't help.

The Bionic Penis

Even the man who is impotent for incurable physical reasons can receive effective treatment today. In fact, there is no cause for a man to remain impotent for any reason unless health or choice precludes surgery: psychological impotence can be treated with therapy; physical impotence can be treated with penile implants. One implant device is so lifelike and natural that no one except the man who has it and his doctor need know that it is artificial.

The inflatable penile prosthesis is the closest thing to a bionic penis that technology has produced and is far more sophisticated than most artificial limbs. It is composed of two tubes that are inserted into the penis, a small pump that is placed inside the scrotum next to the right testicle, and a reservoir that is positioned in the lower abdomen (see diagram).

As shown in the first diagram, the reservoir is implanted underneath the abdominal muscles. Tubings run from there down to the pump, which rests in the scrotum next to the testicles, then into the cylinders, which are threaded into the penis. The system is filled with fluid.

Do you know how much blood it takes to cause an erection? Take a guess. . . Two tablespoons? A pint?

A normal erection takes between fifty and seventy cubic centimeters of blood, which is four to six tablespoons full.

The fluid in the reservoir tubing and pump does the work ordinarily done by your blood. When the fluid remains in the reservoir, the penis looks limp and natural. (See second diagram.) When an erection is desired, the man or his partner grasps the pump through the skin of the scrotum, and works it gently. Fluid is diverted from the reservoir into the tubing in the penis. The more fluid that is pumped, the more erect the penis becomes. He can then have intercourse for as long as he likes. When done, the pump is squeezed in another direction, the fluid is shunted back into the reservoir and the penis deflates.

The idea of a mechanically assisted penis still provokes giggles and off-color comments. Yet, none of those making the remarks would hesitate to make use of the best possible artificial leg available if their own limb was lost. Unfortunately, our attitude toward our sexual anatomy is not as sensible. The implant is often thought of as frivolous or elective.

If you lose a limb, you don't hesitate to get an artificial one. If you have a cataract operation, you will wear contacts gratefully. Yet because of some prejudice against taking sex problems seriously, doctors tend to think that nothing needs to be done for an organically impotent man. The fact is, there are at least two possible solutions to the problem:

1. Alternative forms of sexual gratification that can be learned and enjoyed if the penis is unable to be erect.

2. Implantation of a prosthesis (there are several different types, including plastic rods that are semibendable).

Incidentally, the man with a penis implant continues to feel exactly as he felt before he lost the ability to be erect. If he was able to have an orgasm prior to the surgery, he can still do so after the operation. Most impotent men still have the biological capacity to ejaculate whether they do so or not. Some impotent men ejaculate regularly through a flaccid penis.

Many physicians have not heard of either NPT monitoring or the inflatable implant. Those who have often don't mention them to a male patient unless he specifically asks about such devices. Some doctors simply assume the patient wouldn't want a penis implant, is too old to be interested, or would not be able to afford one. Indeed, it costs about the same amount as a second car (and doesn't use gas).

Implant Considerations

There is one difficulty to consider regarding the semirigid prostheses: A sixty-five-year-old male, statistically, has about a 60 to

THE CANDIDATES

Potential candidates for the penile prosthesis include patients with a wide range of etiologies that contribute to erectile impotence. To date, patients with diabetes, spinal cord injury, peripheral vascular disease, profound anemia and circulatory insufficiencies, post surgical (rectal and prostatic) impotence and injuries to the urethra and pelvic nerves have been successfully treated.

SUCCESSFUL IMPLANTS

The American Medical Systems inflatable penile prosthesis has been employed since 1973 to restore volitional control of the erectile process in men ranging in age from 19 to 83 years old.

Over 55 institutions in the United States, Canada, Western Europe and South America have already been involved in AMS penile prosthetic implants.

THE RESERVOIR

Constructed of silicone elastomer, the reservoir is a storage compartment for the fluid used in the device hydraulic system. Implanted under the muscles of the abdomen, the reservoir is in a protected position where the patient is unaware of its presence. Radioopaque fluid in the reservoir chamber enables easy, concise radiologic analysis of post operative prosthesis function and facilitates follow-up study.

THE CYLINDERS

The inflatable cylinders are placed in a parallel fashion in the penis after making an incision in the tunica albuginea of each corpus cavernosum. Because surgical placement of the cylinders occurs at an abdominal incision, it is not necessary to make an incision in the penis itself. American Medical Systems provides the surgeon with cylinders in a range of sizes to fit varying anatomical requirements. When emptied, the cylinders collapse to guard against tissue erosion and do not interfere with urinary function.

THE PUMP

The bulb shaped pump hangs loosely inside the scrotum and is connected to the cylinders and the reservoir by silicone elastomer tubing. Repeated pumping causes fluid to travel from the reservoir through the tubing to the cylinders which expand and cause erection. A pressure point release valve in the lower portion of the bulb permits fluid to vacate the cylinders, thereby returning the penis to a flaccid state. Since the pressure point is small and the pump is freely movable inside the scrotum, accidental release or loss of erection does not occur.

EASY TO CONTROL

The patient can easily operate and control the prosthesis with no difficulty or discomfort. Its simple design enables patients with limited manual dexterity to operate the prosthesis successfully. The prosthesis does not interfere with or hamper normal physical activity or exercise.

The inflatable penile prosthesis for treatment of erectile impotence

The American Medical Systems inflatable penile prosthesis has been designed to restore sexual function in males suffering from erectile impotence. The prosthesis offers the advantages of volitional patient control to make the penis erect or flaccid, and greatly reduces the risk of tissue perforation commonly associated with "semi-rigid" or "constant erection" type products. The AMS inflatable prosthesis is completely implantable, cosmetically undetectable after surgery and doesn't interfere with the process of orgasm.

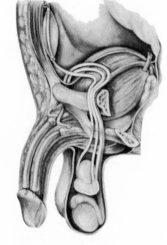

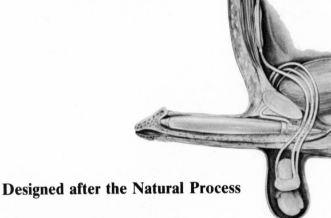

Designed after the Natural Process

The unique yet simple principle of operation of the AMS inflatable penile prosthesis mimics the natural action of the erection process. The miniature hydraulic system of the device transfers fluid to subcutaneously implanted silicone elastomer cylinders. This fluid transfer process causes the cylinders of the prosthesis to fill and expand, creating a suitable full girth erection. When an erection is no longer desired the patient activates the device deflation mechanism to return the penis to a normal flaccid state.

70 percent chance of needing prostate surgery during the next ten years of his life. If he has a hard implant, one that doesn't deflate, the device must be taken out to allow the prostate surgery or the doctor has to go in through the bottom, behind the scrotum and the rectum. So, the hard implants can provide complications that the inflatables do not. The inflatable implant, however, occasionally has mechanical failures or springs a leak.

Premature Ejaculation

Premature ejaculation is a sexist term, one that is unfair to the many men it has made miserable. If the man has an orgasm too fast, we call him a premature ejaculator. If he takes a long time to have an orgasm, we call him virile. The rules for women are reversed! If a woman has an orgasm too fast, that is wonderful. If she takes too long, she is considered frigid. This is an arbitrary definition imposed by man on human nature. The same biological function is defined in the opposite way, depending on whether you happen to be a man or a woman.

I find all the present definitions of premature ejaculation most unsatisfactory. I do not have one I am very pleased with to suggest as a replacement. Common sense, however, will suffice. A brief analysis of other definitions of premature ejaculation may provide some perspective.

The traditional definition of premature ejaculation used to be any man who ejaculated in less than a minute. This definition didn't make too many women happy because even one minute of thrusting is usually not long enough for most women. On the other hand, most men were happy with that definition because the majority could wear "I'm not a premature ejaculator" buttons. Masters and Johnson define premature ejaculation as any man who, more than 50 percent of the time, ejaculates before his partner reaches orgasm, assuming that she is capable of having orgasms. This definition is more realistic but impractical for the single man who has several or a series of relationships. It may define him as a premature ejaculator in one and not a premature ejaculator in another. And, what about the partners who fake orgasm?

Another well-known therapist has defined premature ejaculation as any man who ejaculates when he doesn't want to. That makes almost every man a premature ejaculator because once a man is past the point of ejaculatory inevitability, every man will ejaculate whether he wants to or not.

One man came to therapy for treatment of premature ejaculation although he was not a premature ejaculator by Dr. Master's definition. Although this patient was ejaculating within twenty to thirty seconds, his wife was able to reach orgasm easily in fifteen seconds. She was not only happy with the speed of his ejaculation, she preferred it that way because she was able to, in her words, "stay in control of the situation" and end sex whenever she wanted to. He, on the other hand, wanted to increase his staying power so that he would experience more pleasure for a longer period of time. Thirty seconds wasn't long enough for him.

In the Eye of the Beholder

Premature ejaculation is a very subjective concept. Men who can thrust steadily for half an hour have come to see me, concerned that they are premature ejaculators because their partner hasn't reached her orgasm. Or, they fear that she is used to men with more sexual stamina.

To be sexually secure, a man needs to feel that he has some degree of ejaculatory control. He needs to be able to enjoy sexual activity for a leisurely period of time without fearing that he will ejaculate before he has an opportunity to penetrate. Once he has inserted, he needs to trust that he will be able to savor the experience and enjoy it without ejaculating before he has a chance to be aware of what he is doing. It is nice if he can pay attention to his sexual feelings, rather than struggle to repress them for fear he might enjoy himself so much he will have an orgasm too soon.

He also needs to feel secure that he will last long enough to satisfy the "average" woman.

While women's needs vary tremendously, a minute is usually not enough. More than ten or fifteen minutes of continuous thrusting, even with adequate lubrication, will cause most women to become sore and uncomfortable. Men who aim for half an hour or an hour of sexual stamina can become torture chambers for many women. They strut about proudly, content with their accomplishments, while she is soaking in a sitz bath to relieve the pain. He says, "I can't understand what you're complaining about. Most women would be delighted that I last so long." It is hard for a woman to tell them differently, because such men are convinced that they are right.

Ejaculatory Security

Premature ejaculation is important to the man and the woman for several reasons. Most men tend to lose interest in continuing sexual participation after ejaculation. It is more effort and less enjoyable for them to continue touching immediately following orgasm. Women, on the other hand, do not react this way. After an orgasm, they usually enjoy continuing and can have more orgasms.

A man's ability to control his sexual reflexes is important to his self-image. A man with impotence or rapid ejaculation may feel as distressed as a woman with small breasts. His erection is a symbol of his sexual identity, his masculinity. It isn't the most important thing about him (even if he thinks so), but it is very hard to live without.

Premature ejaculation varies in degree. In its most severe form, a man ejaculates the moment he becomes aroused and is unable to consummate a relationship or have children except through artificial insemination. At the other end of the spectrum is the man who wishes he could last longer. This person isn't quite sure whether or not he is a premature ejaculator. He suspects that the women he is with would prefer him to last longer, and is vaguely troubled by sexual insecurities.

The Knee-Jerk Reflex

To demonstrate how premature ejaculation can be made worse, sit on a bench with your legs dangling loosely over the side. Have someone tap your knee reflexes about one centimeter below your kneecap. Notice the intensity of the reflexes in your legs. Then, cup the fingers of both hands together and pull as hard as you can in opposite directions. While you are pulling, have someone tap your knee reflexes again. You will discover that when you have muscle tension on your arms those knee reflexes are often two to three times as strong as when your arms are relaxed. Check the reflexes again without the muscle tension. Your brain says to your knees, "Someone is tapping your reflexes." However, since your brain knows that you are really not about to fall down, and don't have to correct your balance very dramatically, it tells your knee not to jerk very hard. On the other hand, with muscle tension on your arm, the pathway from your knees to your brain is short-circuited and the gray cells don't interpret the tap on your knee properly. Your knee is not told that you are not losing your balance, so it jerks powerfully—as though you were actually falling down.

Flip Over, Not Out

So what does this have to do with premature ejaculation? Orgasmic response is a reflex of a similar kind. When you're lying passively on your back with pleasant things being done to you, there is ample opportunity to think, evaluate, qualify your biological responses, and edit them in ways you are not even aware. When you are in the astride position, on top, your muscles are more tense (somewhat the way they were when you were pulling on your hands), and your body is more likely to react than to think. This is when the short-circuiting process occurs.

In the case of the premature ejaculator, he is likely to ejaculate more quickly when on top with weight and tension on his arms than when lying on his back. So, what is undesirable for premature ejaculators can be desirable for a woman who wants to become one. The female astride position, which is more conducive to the woman's orgasm (because of the vigorous muscle action it calls for on her part), is the better position for the premature ejaculator as well.

If you have a fast man and a slow woman, flip over. It may help.

The Gravity of It All

A patient of mine was puzzlingly resistant when, in the course of therapy, I suggested he and his wife use the female astride position. His wife could only have an orgasm in that position, yet he usually refused to have sex with her that way. He had no problems with impotence or premature ejaculation, but—as it turned out—he firmly believed that if he was on his back all the blood would run out of his penis and he would lose his erection. He knew it for a fact, because "it had happened once." The power of suggestion again.

In summary, if you think you are a premature ejaculator, you may or may not be. Even if you aren't, you still have a problem of sexual insecurity to sort out in your mind, sometimes with the help of a therapist or counselor. If you are indeed a premature ejaculator who ejaculates before penetration or with just a few thrusts, then you need to decide on your priorities and invest in a little sexual satisfaction rather than that second car or next summer's vacation.

Treatment

As a premature ejaculator, your inability to relate to a woman sexually will inhibit your ability to relate to her well emotionally and may impair the possibilities of intimate meaningful relationships—perhaps for the rest of your life. Don't wait to do something about it. Even if you have waited "too long," which you probably have, it is never too late.

Premature ejaculation is one of the most easily treated of all sexual dysfunctions. With such techniques as talk therapy, stress reduction tactics, and the squeeze technique, a well-qualified therapist can reverse a long-standing problem in a few months—or even in weeks, depending on the form of therapy used. If you decide to live with the problem, be sure it is the choice you want to make.

Ejaculatory Incompetence

Some men have quite a different problem: although they get and maintain erections, it can take from thirty to seventy-five minutes of continuous thrusting to reach orgasm—and some cannot ejaculate no matter how long they are engaged in intercourse.

This is called ejaculatory incompetence. Your mind is filled with enough eroticism to maintain an erection, but not enough to have an orgasm. Some men with this problem have spent most of their lives trying to slow down their orgasm and got so good at it that now they can't hurry up.

Without the ability to turn oneself inward and focus on feelings, ejaculation is more difficult, especially if you are watching your partner instead, or being overly concerned about your performance. There are also some fears of performance involved with ejaculatory incompetence.

Ejaculatory incompetence is a relatively rare sexual dysfunction. These men cannot ejaculate with intercourse. There are some sociologic principles related to ejaculatory incompetence: eight of ten men with the problem are Jewish. It may, however, be a much more common situation than it appears just by looking at the therapeutic population, because people with that difficulty oftentimes don't need or want therapy, particularly if their women like it. Many of these males have partners who are multiply orgasmic. If they consider it a sexual problem, it doesn't bother either one of them enough to come in for treatment.

Some men and women who have this difficulty are troubled by it. In fact, women react just as they do to impotence: feeling inadequate, unattractive, or rejected.

Treatment

As with impotence, most men who cannot ejaculate in the vagina are able to do so with masturbation. (Remember that most impotent men can masturbate without problems.) This form of ejaculatory incompetence is psychological, and responds to the same techniques used in treating psychological impotence.

If the ejaculatory difficulty is due to medical causes, ejaculation will not occur under any circumstances. In this case a medical evaluation is necessary.

Before Seeking Treatment

The sexual problems men experience that were virtually untreatable not so many years ago can usually be cured by modern methods. Unfortunately, most men who are impotent, premature ejaculators, or who have ejaculatory incompetence react by stopping all touching. Because their penis is on strike, they no longer hold, cuddle, caress, or enter ino any alternative form of sexual activity. They are deprived of physical intimacy by choice, not by circumstance.

Explore your value system and discover what alternative forms of sexual activity are within it. Then put them into practice. You will be amazed how far you can go on your own. Your sexual pleasure and participation will return even if your erection doesn't. If the problem isn't physical, your erection has a good chance of returning too.

It is necessary to lighten up a bit, too. Don't be so deadly serious. Bring your sense of humor and become a little vulnerable. Share your fears and watch them disappear.

CHAPTER 13

Your Body — Knowledge Is Power

What You Don't Know Can Hurt You

You would be surprised how many women have never looked at their own genitals. Most men have looked at their own. But few men have seen a woman's genitals in the daylight. Granted, they're a little harder to find than those of a man, but women are resourceful and persistent in other areas. Have you ever watched a little girl try to see the beautiful ribbon on her ponytail? She will circle in front of a mirror to catch a glimpse of a part of her that is hard to see, until her mother gives her a hand mirror and shows her how to use it. Now she can admire the back of her head. Curiosity succeeds.

The Mirror Please

During a physical examination, I routinely use a mirror to demonstrate the various parts of a woman's external and internal genital anatomy. One patient, a nurse, exclaimed: "Oh, you don't need to do any of that. I know where everything is." I replied, "Even if it is information you already know, I prefer to go through the procedure because then I know what you know and you know what I know. There is no room for error."

That's Some Freckle!

When we were done she said, "I am amazed! See this dark spot over here? I always thought that was my clitoris." She had mistaken it for a rather unusually placed but prominent beauty mark.

Of you women who have looked at your own genitals on the outside, how many of you have seen your cervix? Any of you? A few. That is hard to do by yourself. When the doctor says that you have cervicitis, what does that mean? If he says you have dermatitis you can look at it. You may not know what it is but you can see it.

How many of you have asked your doctor to set up a mirror and show you? Many physicians are now providing the opportunity for you to see what it is they're talking about.

In the "old days with the big drape," when the doctor came in to do the pelvic, he disappeared behind his tent. When he talked to you it was a muffled, distant sound. He could sneak out of the room without being seen, before telling you what was wrong or giving you a chance to ask questions.

Become an Expert

Because the woman's anatomy is more subtle than that of a man, it takes more effort to become familiar with it. A certain amount of knowledge about your body and disease is essential to preserving your life and health. You may be surprised at how much you can learn. You don't need four years of medical school to understand diabetes as well as most physicians. For each disease process that must be studied in medical school, doctors receive an hour or two of lecture and spend a few hours or days reading. You can do this too, and it could save your life. It will certainly improve the quality of your health. Don't let the technical terms confuse you. Buy an hour of your favorite physician's time, then say "I want you to explain this problem or disease to me with as much detail as you can possibly give using layman's terms, then recommend whatever books I should read to understand the matter thoroughly." Some physicians may be reluctant, because it is an unusual request, but the majority will accommodate you.

Don't Stop There

If you suspect that something is physically wrong and your doctor says "I can't find anything. There is no problem," don't stop there. Continue your search until you get some satisfactory answers. Above all, don't wait until the problems are so enormous that they cannot be ignored. That is like waiting until you have a stroke to reduce the stress in your life. Earlier is better.

Genital Rules of Order

Following are several general rules that are important to keep in mind.

Intercourse should be painless!   This means *no pain at all*— not even a little bit. Numerous patients, both men and women, have come to see me about pain of varying intensity, telling me that they didn't think anything was wrong because, "Pelvic exams have always hurt and I thought that intercourse was supposed to be painful." One man said, "It hurts a little when I ejaculate, but it's nothing. It feels so good, it's worth it." He had ignored the discomfort for many years until he started becoming impotent, which was no coincidence. His mind wasn't listening, but his penis was. It was refusing to participate because ejaculation hurt.

If there is pain, something is wrong!   The discomfort may not be very serious, but ignoring it can be.

If, as a woman, you are not lubricating enough and intercourse hurts, better do something about it before you have a real problem. Add a little extra lubrication and have him ease up on the thrusting, or you will become irritated and tender. If that happens, you won't be able to have intercourse comfortably for quite a while and you could end up with a vaginal or a bladder infection. Some women object "I don't want to use anything artificial." You use makeup, don't you? Hand lotion? Would you rather have pain and disease? It's your decision.

Vaginal discharges are not innocent!   When not taken care of they can lead to severe problems. A low-grade, not too annoying vaginal discharge can cause irritation around the opening to the bladder, and with very little encouragement, an infection can move into the bladder and from there into the kidneys. Bladder infections are painful but usually are not a serious threat to your health—if caught and treated early. On the other hand, kidney problems, which are only one step beyond a bladder infection, can be life-threatening. The female genital parts are closely interrelated, both in health and in disease. A minor problem in one area can lead to major problems in other areas.

There are normal innocent secretions that vary in consistency, volume, and color. These secretions don't itch, cause pain, or have a foul odor, and they don't require treatment.

Don't hesitate to get a second opinion! As a man, if you complain to your urologist, internist, or family practitioner about a discharge or burning at the tip of your penis, discomfort with ejaculation, impotence, or premature ejaculation—and the treatment seems ineffective—don't simply let it go. As a woman, if there is pain, discharge, or any other symptoms that are not responding to treatment, get a second opinion, a third opinion, or whatever number seem needed to resolve the problem. Keep searching until you get an answer, and if possible, a solution.

Be helpful to your doctor! If you are having a hard time discussing your sexual problem, imagine how your doctor feels, especially if he or she is much older than you. It should not be this way, but at this time, that is often the was it is. Did you know that not until the 1960s did any American medical school offer a course on human sexuality? Physicians who graduated before then received no training in this area unless they took postgraduate training courses. Even now, in the 1980s, in over 80 percent of our medical schools, courses in human sexuality are elective, not required. So, don't assume your doctor is knowledgeable in sexual problems. Don't be afraid to ask questions and don't be satisfied until you get the answers.

Pelvic examinations aren't supposed to hurt! How many of you women have had a pelvic exam that hurt? If so, you are probably enduring some unnecessary discomfort. If the pelvic exam hurts, there is either something wrong with you or with the doctor's technique; there are no other reasons for a pelvic exam to be painful. However, most women are stoic, refined, and don't tell their physician that it hurts. Moreover, most doctors still are male. Male gynecologists don't have vaginas, so they don't know what it feels like to have a pelvic exam and never will. If you don't tell him when it is uncomfortable, your doctor is never going to know. If, instead (like most women) you lie there with an ''oh well, pelvics ought to hurt'' attitude, your doctor's technique will never improve, and some important problems may go undetected! You would be amazed how many physicians alter their technique of giving proctoscopies (rectal exams, with a long instrument) after they have had their first one. Don't hesitate to say, ''Ouch, that hurts,'' or ''I'm uncomfortable,'' and you will receive a more gentle exam.

The Physical Examination

When does the woman need a physical examination? There are several situations when one should be done:

- If you experience pain with intercourse.
- If there is an absence of lubrication when you are sexually aroused.
- If you have an excessive discharge.
- If there is a strong vaginal odor.
- If you need reassurance: ''My vagina is numb, my genitals aren't normal'' etc.
- If you are unable to consummate your marriage.

Painful Intercourse Can Be Life-Threatening

Serious disease (and even suicide) can sometimes be the result. Recently, a patient came to me for help. Four years earlier she had developed such severe pain with intercourse that she couldn't participate. At that time, the gynecologist who examined her said there was nothing wrong. He suggested she see a psychiatrist. She didn't.

During the next several months, she became progressively more depressed, and allowed her appearance to deteriorate. She refused to leave the house, withdrew from her husband and her friends, and often would not even get out of bed in the morning. One day she slit her wrists. She was transferred from the emergency room to a mental hospital, where she remained for six months, treated with antidepressants and shock therapy. Eventually, she was returned home on medication.

A few years later, she and her husband separated. Amazingly enough, during the four years she had been unable to have intercourse, no one had given her a second pelvic exam. By the time she consulted me, she was coping better with day-to-day living, and had determined to try one more time to discover and treat the cause of her pain.

A pelvic examination revealed the location of her pain, but we were not able to diagnose it without further studies. She agreed to undergo a laparoscopy (an exploratory surgery); it revealed spots of endometriosis, a common pelvic disease, which were then cauterized (burned away). The pain disappeared. One year later she was back together with her husband, expecting a child, delighted, and free from pain with intercourse.

If her physician had not been so quick to conclude it was a mental problem, the physical problem might have been discovered much sooner. Had she been treated surgically earlier, she would have been spared an incredible amount of pain and grief.

It Isn't "All in Your Head"

A woman came to me recently complaining that after every intercourse episode she developed a painful bladder infection, a rather common problem. Sex had become so uncomfortable that she could not participate at all. Most of the doctors she went to told her that it was a psychological problem and referred her for psychoanalysis—which may have helped her to better understand herself, but which did nothing for her painful bladder.

The fact is, her four sisters all have chronic bladder problems, so she may be genetically predisposed to this type of difficulty. Medical problems are sometimes misdiagnosed as psychological.

One must not assume that pain with intercourse is "in your head." The trouble may have started there, but by the time you experience the pain, you have some sort of associated physical problem. It is true that many diseases are emotionally induced: high blood pressure, heart attacks, and ulcers, for example. In such cases doctors sometimes make the mistake of treating only the physical problem. However, even if they do refer the ulcer sufferer to a psychiatrist, they first provide medication for the physical problem. A doctor faced with a person who is complaining of painful intercourse, however, will often send that person to a psychiatrist *without* diagnosing or treating the physical problem at all.

We all know that while ulcers are stress-induced, there is also a hole in your stomach or intestines. Similarly, heart disease is stress-induced, but the blockages in your arteries are very real. Painful intercourse can be stress-induced also, but there is a physical problem too—which is responsible for the pain you experience.

Most Cases of Painful Intercourse Are Not Stress-Induced

As you can well imagine, painful intercourse will produce stress. Thus, the physical problem develops into a psychological problem. A woman unable to have intercourse will be disturbed, upset, unhappy, and feel abnormal. That is perfectly appropriate under the circumstances.

When the symptom of painful intercourse exists, assume that the problem is physical until proven otherwise. (Common medical causes of painful intercourse are listed in Table II.) Although there are always psychological factors involved when there is pain, there is a physical lesion somewhere. The cause could be vaginismus, a tiny herpes blister, or a sore the size of a paper cut. The barely seen paper cut on your finger hurts a lot. A paper cut at the opening to your vagina may not be seen by the gynecologist; but you know something's wrong—the pain is real.

Use a mirror to inspect your genitals. Try to find the sore spot with your own finger; and during the pelvic examinations, show the gynecologist where it hurts. If you can't reach inside far enough, then be sure the physician finds the area that stings, burns, or aches. Let the doctor know when his (or her) finger has located the painful area, and be sure it is the same kind of pain you feel with intercourse.

TABLE II
COMMON CAUSES OF PAINFUL INTERCOURSE

Cause	Symptoms	Treatment
1. • Mechanical irritation • Lack of lubrication:	• Pain on insertion. • Varies throughout sex depending on degree of lubrication present. • Often gets worse during sex. • Disappears if artificial lubrication is used.	• Artificial lubrication: KY Jelly or other water-soluble, nonallergenic substance (no Vaseline). • Abstain from intercourse until symptoms are gone.
2. Constipation	• Pain with deep thrusting, constant or intermittent.	• Stool softener or shallow thrusting.
3. Vaginismus	• Burning or tearing sensation. • Pelvic exams are always painful. • Constant discomfort during intercourse. • Pain at opening especially during intercourse.	• Painless dilation and psychotherapy.
4. Cervical or uterine discomfort	• Does not disappear if artificial lubrication is used. • Pain with deep thrusting. • Intermittent.	• Appropriate medical treatment. • Altered angle of thrusting.
5. Cystitis	• Burning on urination. • Frequency of urination. • Blood in urine.	• Antibiotics. • No intercourse until symptoms are gone.
6. Herpes	• Pain.	• No intercourse during active outbreak. Acyclovir.

Cause	Symptoms	Treatment
7. Vaginal infection	• Pain. • Discharge. • Itching.	• Specific medicine for specific infection. • Treatment of both partners. • Abstain from intercourse during symptoms.
8. Endometriosis	• Intermittent pain with deep thrusting (constant if uterus tilted).	• Hormones or surgery.
9. Tumors or masses	• Pain with deep thrusting. • Intermittent or constant.	• Surgery or altered position.

Vaginismus

Vaginismus is the most common pain problem that is sent to the psychiatrist without a proper medical diagnosis. Vaginismus is an involuntary contraction of the muscles near the vaginal opening. It can be caused by either a physical or a psychological problem. The contraction can be so severe that it makes penetration impossible, or it can be mild, making penetration merely somewhat uncomfortable. The discomfort is usually located about one-half to one inch into the vagina.

Vaginismus is commonly misdiagnosed because there is little to see during physical examination. A doctor, using a speculum, can wrench the muscles involved apart, and conclude that everything is normal.

A woman who had seen eighteen gynecologists came to see me for treatment. The last doctor finally referred her to sex therapy. His letter to me went something like this:

"I have examined this patient and I can find absolutely nothing wrong. The pelvic examination was absolutely normal—except for the screaming. I hope you can help her."

Vaginismus is an involuntary muscle contraction. Where else in your body does this happen? If you tighten your calf muscles on purpose, they don't hurt; but if the muscles contract involuntarily, they hurt a lot. That is a cramp. Stretching out a cramped muscle hurts, burns, or tears.

The patient with vaginismus usually describes the discomfort as a tearing or burning sensation, rather than a tightness. If the condition is severe, the pain which occurs during attempted penetration generally does not disappear, but remains persistent.

Many women will complain of a slight burning sensation during intercourse, which they disregard on the assumption that it is just lack of lubrication. In fact, it is actually a mild degree of vaginismus and, because the woman doesn't say it hurts, is not likely to be detected during a routine pelvic exam.

What is the difference between vaginismus and vaginitis?

Vaginitis is an infection. Vaginismus is an involuntary muscle spasm. They are not related.

There are several causes of vaginismus. One of the most common is painful intercourse due to some other physical problem. Example: A woman has a tilted uterus, with endometriosis (abnormal tissue growth) and consequently feels pain with deep thrusting. She doesn't have vaginismus yet, and continues to have intercourse, even though it hurts. Eventually, her body will talk to her, by contracting the vaginal muscles. It is essentially saying: "Look, self, that hurts. Don't do it anymore. If you haven't got the sense to stop and find out what the problem is, I'm going to make it hurt more so you'll have to stop." Physical pain with intercourse from any cause eventually will result in vaginismus if that pain is allowed to continue untreated.

Another cause of vaginismus is certain kinds of physical discipline. In some women—particularly dancers, gymnasts, and others who exercise the muscles of their lower body—the muscles around the opening to the vagina hypertrophy (enlarge), just as other muscles do when a person does pull-ups or push-ups. The vaginal muscles can get so strong that they create a physical barrier to penetration. Although these women have no psychological or medical problem, they may develop vaginismus severe enough to prevent penetration.

The other major cause of vaginismus is psychological. Women raised in a very strict, "sex is sin, don't touch yourself," environment can be severely affected, although there has been no sign of it before they attempted intercourse. Vaginismus, by the way, is one of the most common causes of an unconsummated marriage.

What is the cure for vaginismus?

Normally, a combination of limited psychotherapy and supervised dilation procedures works quite successfully. The problem can usually be resolved with daily sessions for two weeks, or one or two sessions weekly for two or three months. Even the most severe cases can usually be treated in that time frame.

If you hand a package of dilators to a woman with vaginismus and say, "Go home and use these," you will probably never see her again. Once she sees the larger sizes she gets discouraged and quits.

Dilators alone are an incredibly ineffective technique. Talk therapy alone is not enough either. If you try to talk a woman out of her vaginismus, the process is much the same as if you tried to talk someone out of an ulcer. Sure, the problem is stress-induced, but—as with an ulcer—if you don't also treat the ulcer medically, your chances of success are low. When a person has developed vaginismus, the treatment must use both psychological and physiological means. The combined effort is effective and rapid, and the disease rarely recurs.

*How to Tell the Difference Between a Normal
Discharge and an Infection*

A doctor I once knew treated vaginal infections this way: "It is just a little cold in your vagina, dear, it will go away."

Women's natural secretions are difficult to study because so many abnormal discharges (infections) interfere. We do know that, from the time they are babies, women have a vaginal discharge. The amount varies from almost nonexistent to abundant, the consistency can be anything from thin and watery to thick and mucoid, and the color ranges from clear and transparent to opaque.

An abnormal discharge smells somewhat foul or fishy and may cause itching. The color may be yellow, green, or white. If you go to your physician with an unusual odor, a colored discharge, or discomfort and itching and he or she tells you there is nothing wrong, ask the doctor to take some cultures for bacteria and yeast, or else get a second opinion.

Help Stamp Out Yeast Infections!

Yeast infections have so many aliases that a patient can think she has had many different diseases. Candida, monilia, fungus, and yeast are synonyms (like Tylenol and acetamenophen mean the same thing). A yeast infection is also referred to by doctors as a "cottage cheese" or "curdish white" infection because of the color and consistency of the discharge. There is sometimes a musty or yeasty odor. The most prominent symptoms are itching and irritation. A good rule of thumb: when irritative symptoms predominate, think yeast until proven otherwise. Pain with intercourse is not usual, but occurs occasionally.

Most yeast infections are caused by self-inoculation. Yeasts normally live in the rectum and intestinal tract in both men and women. The woman's rectum and vagina are very close together—very poor plumbing planning—but healthy bacteria normally living in the vagina usually crowd out any foreign intruders. Most of the "good guys" are lactobacilli, microorganisms found in yogurt. Thus some women have considered spooning yogurt into their vagina. (I do not recommend this approach. The yogurt is cold and it is terribly awkward to get the spoon in and out.)

Some doctors prescribe lactobacillus capsules, to help a woman's vagina fight against foreign intruders. It would be a good idea, except that the intestinal juices digest and dissolve the bacteria long before they can get to the vagina.

When You Are at Risk

If you are taking antibiotics, you are more likely to get a yeast infection, because, although the drugs kill off the "bad" bacteria, they also kill off the "good" bacteria—and don't affect the yeast at all. The yeast can then grow without any competition.

Pregnant women and those on the birth control pill are more susceptible to yeast infections. And yeast, like most other organisms, grows well on sugars, so diabetics (who have more sugar in their systems) get yeast infections more easily. Such organisms also grow on blood, so women are more prone to getting yeast infections during menstrual periods.

The Ping-Pong Effect

A not widely publicized fact about yeast infections—and one of the reasons that women go through chronic persistent yeast infections without relief—is the ping-pong effect. Men harbor yeast in their ejaculate and are asymptomatic (it doesn't bother them). The woman will be fine as long as she is on the medication. As soon as she stops—if the man still has the yeast in his system—the women will get another infection. Until recently, there has been no pill or medication to help the man get rid of what he is carrying, so there were only two ways to prevent the ping-pong effect: wearing a condom during his wife's treatment, or abstaining from intercourse, giving his natural immune system an opportunity to clear the organism. Now there is an oral medication called Nizoral that is effective.

What is the most common source of yeast infections?

Self-contamination from the woman's own rectum. When a woman lubricates or sweats it is impossible to keep vaginal and rectal organisms separate. The only reason that she doesn't get a yeast infection every time she has intercourse is because, as we mentioned earlier, she has healthy bacteria protecting her vagina and a good immune system that wipes out any yeast creatures that may wander in.

The second most common way to get such an infection is to have intercourse with a man who carries the yeast in his ejaculate. There is no way to tell if he does or doesn't because he almost invariably has no symptoms.

Does yeast ever appear visibly on a man?

In a small percentage of cases, a man will get a small, pimply rash (sometimes itchy or tender) on the head or shaft of his penis. This condition is often not recognized as a yeast infection by the patient or the physician. Rashes around the rectum or scrotum (jock itch) are usually yeast, and can cause a vaginal infection in a woman, too, if abundant enough.

A note about anal intercourse is in order at this point. Germs from the anal area, if they invade the vagina, can cause an infection. Therefore, if you have anal intercourse followed by vaginal intercourse, infection-producing yeast, as well as other undesirables (E. Coli, strep faecalis, etc.), will most certainly be carried from the anal canal to the vaginal area.

There may be other ways in which a yeast infection can get started. For example, fungus and yeasts go into spore (inactive) forms, so the "borrowed bathing suit" theory of how a vaginal infection develops could be true in this instance. Women may get it from their baby's diaper rash or partner's jock itch. It is thought that stress can change a woman's vaginal chemistry, making her more susceptible to infection.

Does oral sex contribute to yeast infections?

It can, but probably doesn't very often. *Occasionally* people do carry yeast in their mouths, but they also have many other germs there. Your rectum is consistently a lot closer than anyone's mouth and a lot more contaminated. Monilia, by the way, is the same organism that causes thrush in little babies. For some reason, adults don't develop thrush in their mouths, so monilia is not a high risk with oral sex.

Yeast infections are usually treated with vaginal suppositories such as Nystatin, Gyne-Lotrimin, and Monistat. Nystatin (Mycolog) ointment or cream can be used externally to soothe the itching and soreness.

For yeast, you should be treated for at least two weeks and then use the medicine again during each menstrual period for three months to prevent the infection from cropping up again soon.

If a yeast infection is persistent in spite of these treatment measures, take Nystatin tablets orally three times a day for a week or two. This medicine will not go into your bloodstream, and therefore won't kill the yeast in your vagina, but will kill the yeast in your gastrointestinal tract, thus cutting down on the population which is available to reinfect you.

Also keep in mind that yeast infections are the same organism responsible for your baby's diaper rash. Exposure to air, heat, and keeping dry will all help.

If you are susceptible to recurrent yeast infections, take preventive measures whenever you are taking antibiotics by inserting an antiyeast suppository at bedtime for as long as you are on the prescription.

There is now a new drug—Nizoral—that can treat yeast infections in women and men. It can be taken by mouth and will treat the vaginal infection as well as the carrier state in men. Most physicians are not yet familiar with it, but the drug is available, and the results are excellent. It makes the use of suppositories and vaginal creams unnecessary in most cases.

Trichomonas

What is trichomonas? Trichomonas is a vaginal infection caused by the protozoan *Trichomonas vaginalis*. It causes a frothy, whitish discharge. It is usually more liquid in consistency than yeast and has a stronger odor.

There seems to be a conspiracy of silence about the source of trichomonas. It does not fly through the air. It is, to the best of everyone's knowledge, a venereally transmitted disease. If a woman suddenly gets trichomonas, either she or her partner has been involved in sex with someone who has it. Perhaps one can get trichomonas from wearing the bathing suit of a friend who has this vaginal infection. I don't know if it is possible, but I do know that no one has ever cultured old bathing suits to answer that question one way or the other.

Trichomonas symptoms may be triggered by the onset of sexual activity, a new partner, or a specific coital event. This is the only vaginitis that by itself commonly causes all three symptoms: irritation, heavy discharge, and bad odor. It does not usually cause painful intercourse, however.

Trichomonas vaginalis is passed from male to female or vice versa. If a doctor tells you you have trichomonas, both you and your mate need to take an oral medication called Flagyl. Antibiotics will not cure you.

An historical perspective: Did you know that, until recently, trichomonas was considered a mental disorder?

Trichomonas was first identified as a type of vaginitis in 1916. In 1943 it was determined to be a venereal disease. Some experts disagreed, insisting that it was a psychological condition. In

1957, utilizing glitter wax and plasticine, researchers elegantly proved that there can be viable trichomonads in toilet splash. However, in the 1960s many doctors still insisted that trichomonas was an emotional problem. In 1959 one paper reported curing a "frigid neurotic" of trichomonas by "a simple plastic enlargement of the introitus" (increasing the size of the opening of the vagina). In another classic perversion of cause and effect, the researcher declared that emotional tension is the most important factor in the recurrence of trichomonal infections. He went on to express surprise that patients wanted to discuss vaginitis with their gynecologist rather than the "real problems" of penis envy and fear of flying.

Then, in 1972, several studies demonstrated the success of Flagyl (a pill) for the cure of trichomonas, and the debate died.

Pity the women turned into nervous wrecks by the wrong diagnosis. *Beware of the tendency in medicine to diagnose as psychosomatic everything that can not be easily understood.*

Gonorrhea

A study done in Sweden involved placing cultures of gonorrhea on porcelain fixtures such as: sinks, light bulbs, door handles, etc. The researchers went back at half-hour and hourly intervals for a period of twenty-four to forty-eight hours to see if they could reculture gonorrhea from those sites. The experiment was an attempt to answer the question, "Can you get gonorrhea from a toilet seat?" They did determine that a porcelain fixture or door handle inoculated with the gonorrhea organism could be recultured up to twenty-four hours later. Now that doesn't mean that, at that point, you would catch the disease. It does say that the absolute statement that you can only get gonorrhea from sex may not always be true.

Gonorrhea may result in a yellowish discharge and bad odor but it is usually asymptomatic in the woman. The man usually has a yellowish discharge from his penis, but not always. There are asymptomatic carriers.

I once had a couple referred to me because the wife had a terrible vaginal reaction every time they had intercourse. The referring physician thought she was allergic to her husband's sperm. (There have been two or three reported cases of women going into anaphylactic shock due to intercourse with a man whose sperm they were allergic to.) The cultures done on her were negative. Her husband had no symptoms of any infection and cultures of his urine and prostatic secretions were also negative. It was not until I cultured his ejaculate (not a common procedure) that we were able to grow an abundant amount of gonorrhea. We were eventually able to culture gonorrhea from her vagina too. They were both treated with penicillin and the problem disappeared.

The treatment of both (or more) partners is a high dosage of penicillin, or penicillin substitute. There are unfortunately some resistant strains, and Pelvic Inflammatory disease (infection in tubes and ovaries) is a common complication.

Beta Strep Vaginitis

Beta strep vaginitis is usually painless and asymptomatic. When symptomatic, however, it feels like a strep throat and can be very painful. There may or may not be much discharge: however, if the vagina and the vulva hurt, intercourse will usually be painful.

B-strep vaginitis is dangerous for several reasons: babies that pass through a vaginal canal with B-strep present sometimes die within the first few days of life; women who have severe B-strep vaginitis can develop the same medical complications that strep throats can cause; and you can give your partner strep throat if he performs cunnilingus, or get strep vaginitis if you have oral sex with someone who has strep throat.

Hemophilus Vaginalis

Irritative symptoms are rare, and the volume of the discharge varies. The main symptom is a bad odor (smells fishy), like walrus breath. Treatment is Flagyl or ampicillin for both partners. It is transmitted through sexual contact, and although men are not symptomatic, both partners need to be treated.

TABLE III
VAGINITIS CHART

Problem	Discharge	Symptoms
Yeast (monilia candida, fungus)	• White. • Curdy, grainy, thick, cottage cheeselike. • Mild to moderate amount.	• Itching (think yeast until proven otherwise). • Burning swollen lips, redness, soreness (looks like diaper rash). • Mild musty odor. • Pain with intercourse
Trichomonas	• Yellowish-white. • Frothy liquid.	• Foul odor. • Heavy discharge. • Some itching.
Gonorrhea	• Yellowish, if present	• Often *none*. • Women can harbor organism for months, even years without knowing it (so can men).
Herpes	• None.	• Sores. • Severe pain.
Hemophilus vaginalis	• Rare. • Grayish.	• Fishy odor. • Usually no pain with intercourse.
Beta strep vaginitis	• Minimal.	• Pain with and without intercourse, or no pain at all.
Chlamydia	• Thin, watery.	• Burning on urination.
Cervicitis	• Yellow or green. • Mucoid. • Thick, copious.	• Significant increase in volume of secretions.

TABLE III (*Continued*)
VAGINITIS CHART

Source	*Treatment*
• Sexual contact or self-inoculation. • More susceptible if diabetic, pregnant, or menstruating. • Taking antibiotics, birth control pills, hormones, steroids.	• Vaginal suppositories or creams like Nystatin, Monistat, Mycelex, Gyne-Lotrimin for two weeks to one month. *Antibiotics don't work.* • Nystatin oral tabs. • Abstain from intercourse or use a condom. • Sitz baths, local heat for comfort. • Continue treatment for next three menstrual periods. • Nizoral orally for self and partner(s).
• Sexual contact.	• Flagyl for self and partner(s).
• Sexual contact.	• Penicillin (or substitute) in high doses. • Partner(s) must be treated.
• Sexual contact.	• No intercourse when sores are present. • Acyclovir.
• Sexual contact.	• Flagyl. • Ampicillin.
• Sexual partner or self-inoculation.	• Penicillin (or substitute).
• Sexual contact.	• Tetracycline.
• Sexual partner or self-inoculation.	• Cautery. • Freezing. • Antibiotics.

Herpes

Herpes is our newest and most formidable venereal disease. It afflicts some 15 to 20 million Americans, and according to the Center for Disease Control in Atlanta, is spreading at epidemic proportions—some 500,000 new cases a year. It is particularly prevalent in white sexually active men and women between the age of twenty-five and thirty-five. It is similar to the cold sore you are all familiar with but occurs on the genitals. Small, painful, recurrent blistery lesions are typical.

The first symptoms of herpes may be tingling or itching. Blisters appear within two to fifteen days. The first episode lasts two to three weeks, subsequent episodes last only five to six days. The episodes are usually more severe in women than men, although sometimes women who have the blisters internally may not even be aware they have them and can unknowingly infect someone else.

Herpes is caused by a virus. Some people are susceptible to it, others have an immune system that protects them. Once transmitted, it sometimes lies dormant for months or years before recurring. Stress often precipitates a recurrence, and oral sex is a contributing factor.

There are two types of herpes—type I and type II. It used to be thought that type I occurred above the waist (cold sores), type II below (genital herpes). That distinction is disappearing. One survey shows that one-third of women under twenty-four who have herpes on their genitals have type I, so avoid kissing, or sexual contact, if you have an active blister anywhere (that includes kissing friends and children).

The psychological effects of herpes can be devastating. Some victims feel like lepers—socially isolated. Most go through a process very much like mourning after they are diagnosed with it.

Lysine, available in most health food stores, taken daily, has been used in an attempt to prevent recurrences.

Until recently, there has been no proven effective treatment for genital herpes. The U.S. Food and Drug Administration has just approved a new drug called acyclovir (trade name Zovirax), which is a local ointment that has shown promising results in the treatment of herpes. It is most useful for the first outbreak. Oral and injectable forms are being tested and are expected to be more effective.

Chlamydia

This is another infection that is sexually transmitted, but testing for this condition is usually not available in physicians' offices or local laboratories. About 3 million Americans are affected. The symptoms are burning on urination and a watery discharge, and it is often confused with gonorrhea. It usually responds to treatment with tetracycline.

How Can You Tell If He or She Is Having an Affair?

All of the above vaginal infections can be venereally transmitted. Yeast infections can be transmitted through intercourse but are most commonly derived from yourself. Herpes, yeast, and beta strep as well as hemophilus can be transmitted through oral sex as well. If you develop any vaginal problem and the physician treats both you and your partner, this means that this condition can be sexually transmitted.

A Sexually Transmitted Disease (STD) is a genital (and other parts of the body too) ailment which you get from someone else—as a result of having sex with that person. Some infections that you can get through sexual activity can also be caused by self-inoculation. Yeast infections are an example.

Understanding the source and the cause of infection can help you prevent them, treat them, and interpret the probabilities of whether your partner is having an affair.

If it is gonorrhea, syphilis, genital herpes, hemophilus vaginalis, trichomonas, or chlamydia, the answer is yes, with the rarest exceptions. Gonorrhea can be contracted from porcelain fixtures. Syphilis can be contracted by kissing someone with a chancre (sore) on his or her lip. Recent evidence on herpes reveals that it can also be recovered from inanimate objects— toilet seats, doorknobs, towels. So there are few absolutes.

If it is B-strep it is possible but not probable.

If it is yeast, it is possible, but far more probable that she developed it on her own.

In general, while there are unusual circumstances other than sex where it is possible to get one of these infections, if a woman gets two or three different ones or frequent recurrences (other than monilia), it is almost certain that she or her spouse is having intercourse with someone else.

Recap

When vaginitis becomes chronic or recurrent, it will negatively affect your sex life—all the way from just causing an inconvenience to making it unwise or impossible to have intercourse.

A trichomonal infection is generally more liquid than yeast. Yeast is renowned for its itching. Any discharge that has a particularly foul odor is probably a bacterial infection, in which bacteria that don't belong in your vagina have overgrown and multiplied. Gonorrhea is usually yellowish, and hemophilus smells fishy. If the discharge is green or any other bizarre color, see a doctor. Refer to Table III for comparison of symptoms.

Cervicitis

Cervicitis is infection and inflammation of the cervix. The symptoms consist of a heavy, mucoid discharge. The sexual partner often has present or past history of urethritis, either gonococcal or "nonspecific" (NSU), but experts disagree on the cause. There may be associated spotting, after intercourse or otherwise. Cervicitis can be asymptomatic (without symptoms) or very prominently symptomatic. The most characteristic symptom is a significant increase in volume of secretions—which are often thick, yellow or green, and/or mucoid. Irritation is rare but can occur. Malodor is rare.

Cystitis

I have found that very few young women are told about cystitis before they get married. Perhaps that is why they are so susceptible to "honeymoon cystitis," an ironic title considering that it is no honeymoon to have this irritating and annoying ailment.

When the male puts his erect penis into the woman's vagina, if he rides high (or thrusts high), as many marriage manuals and sex-how-to-do-it books recommend, he will crush and irritate the bladder opening. (Imagine what it would be like if you took a toothbrush and rubbed it on that sensitive mucous membrane on the inside of your mouth.) Irritation occurs and germs set in. They back up the very short tube (about an inch to an inch and a half long) to the bladder, and usually create a bladder infection. If you feel any burning sensation with urination, frequency, or have other reasons to believe you have an infection there, see your physician for treatment. Don't ignore it. Avoid alcohol, coffee, and drinks with stimulants in them, such as most dark-colored colas; drink a lot of liquids to help irrigate and flush your kidneys and bladder. Treat any vaginal infection that may coexist and predispose you to cystitis.

Some people recommend drinking cranberry juice, an acidifying agent, to help ease cystitis symptoms. The theory is that if you give the urine a higher acid content, you create a more hostile environment for germs. Thus, when the vagina and urine are fairly acidic, they are less likely to get infected.

If you are susceptible to cystitis always urinate before intercourse—which is generally a good idea anyway, because intercourse does not feel good with a full bladder. And, if you urinate immediately following intercourse, even if it is only a teaspoon or two, that will help to flush out any germs.

Refrain from intercourse when you first start noticing some discomfort. During the treatment of a bladder infection (or urethritis) avoid intercourse. Your orgasm (or his) doesn't have to happen with the penis in the vagina. If you continue to have intercourse, you may pay an unnecessarily high price in pain and illness.

Precautions and Treatments

There are several precautions a woman can take to avoid getting vaginal infections and bladder infections:

1. After urination or a bowel movement, wipe from the front to the back with each tissue. The bladder opening comes first, then the opening to the vagina, then the opening to the rectum. The germs in the rectum can cause infection in the vagina; those in the rectum and vagina can cause infections in the bladder. Thus, wiping from the rectum to the front smears all of the infectious organisms over the vulnerable places. Wiping from fore to aft does not do so. Teach your little girls the proper direction to wipe; the constant threat of infection in one of these areas will be greatly reduced by this simple ritual.

Healthy urine is bacteriologically sterile (no germs). In fact, you could drink it and it would not hurt you. When there are germs in it, something is wrong and the result is a burning sensation during urination. Normally, however, urine is pure. The vagina, however, has a conglomerate of healthy germs. The rectum normally has many germs, including yeasts and bacteria capable of causing infection when relocated. Thus, because a woman's rectum and vagina are not far apart, women are more prone than men to be attacked by yeast and bacteria.

2. Wear cotton underpants. Yeasts and other organisms like to live in moist, sweaty places and cotton underpants help prevent this condition from developing by allowing your skin to breathe and your secretions to be absorbed. If you wear pantyhose, be sure they have a cotton crotch.

If your infection has become chronic, or if you get the attacks frequently, there are some additional things you should know:

3. Be sure that your physician is treating the infection with a medicine specifically designed to kill the organism infecting you. Nystatin, Gyne-Lotrimin, and Monistat are specifically for yeast, and won't cure anything else. Flagyl is prescribed for trichomonas and hemophilus; penicillin is for gonorrhea.

4. Avoid intercourse during an active infection time— whether bladder or vaginal. You can have other sexual play and activity, but when your vaginal skin tissues are raw and irritated, or your urinary tract is infected any mechanical friction will delay healing.

If you insist on having intercourse, your husband should use a condom during your treatment period, and perhaps, for a while thereafter to prevent the ping-pong effect. If your problems have been severe, ask a physician to culture your husband's ejaculate for yeast and bacteria to make sure he is clear before resuming intercourse.

5. Take sitz baths and occasional vinegar douches (no more than once or twice a week) for comfort and a soothing effect. Strong unpleasant genital and vaginal odors—unless there is infection involved—come from the bacterial action on the perspiration in the *external* genital area. Cleansing the external area alone is, therefore, usually enough. Too much douching can bring on infections. A douche mechanically irrigates out the good bacteria that you need to protect you against "bad guys." In recent years physicians have advised no douching. This trend is changing. Nonetheless, frequent douching is to be avoided.

6. Women who are susceptible to bladder and yeast infections, or other similar infections, should not use artificial lotions, flavored douches, or scented preparations. Anything that is okay for a baby's skin will be fine on your own. Don't use potions that may have chemicals in them or that could be harsh on your skin.

7. If you need lubrication, use a surgical jelly such as K-Y Jelly or Lubifax or WD40. Do not use Vaseline.

8. Keep a box of Wet Ones, or something similar, at the bedside to use after sex so you don't have to get up immediately, if you would rather just lay there.

9. Pay early and prompt attention to any itching or irritation.

With that regimen of treatment, most infections can be cured. This process may appear to involve a lot of effort and inconvenience, but if you have had a year or two of on-and-off-again bouts of infection, itching, and irritation, the process is well worth going through.

Pregnancy

Did any of your doctors talk to you about sex during, before, or after delivery? Did anybody ever say anything other than "no sex"?

Often physicians will say "no sex," meaning no intercourse,

and people deny themselves any touching, orgasms, or sexual contact during this period of time. In some cases, however, your doctor may really mean no orgasms. If your pregnancy is in jeopardy—for example, you've miscarried a number of times—and you want to be extra careful, the doctor may mean no orgasms because the rhythmic and expulsive contractions of the uterus during orgasm may not be desirable and could trigger labor.

If the doctor means no intercourse, that means no penis in the vagina, and no thrusting against the uterus, the cervix, or the baby during the last few weeks of pregnancy.

Ask more specific questions to clarify what you can do and cannot do. The rules keep changing as we learn more. After all, if the restriction is against intercourse but not against having orgasms, you can continue to enjoy sex through partner manipulation or masturbation.

Following delivery (not immediately—wait a week or so), orgasms are good for you. In fact, the standard postdelivery procedure is to tell you to rub your uterus to make it clamp down. (If you're nursing, the uterus will shrink up faster than if you're not because of the hormones circulating in your system.) Orgasms cause the uterus to clamp down and once again become a nice tight little muscle. So, orgasms after delivery will help your uterus bounce back faster. Intercourse may be harmful, however, especially if you have had an episiotomy or a complicated delivery. There are stitches and your tissue has not healed yet.

The main reason for waiting at least six weeks is that the cervix, usually tight and small, is expanded by delivery of a child. It takes time for that cervix to tighten up, and the doctor doesn't want the possibility of any infection backing up into the uterus and fallopian tubes.

However, if you have a Cesarean section, you are capable of having intercourse as soon as you are pain-free, and your doctor gives approval.

Hysterectomy

You'd be surprised how many women have had hysterectomies and don't exactly know what was taken out of them.

A pan hysterectomy involves taking the ovaries, fallopian tubes, and uterus. You're left with a sewn-up space in a vaginal pouch.

A total hysterectomy usually involves taking out just the uterus (the cervix included), leaving the ovaries and the tubes there to continue producing hormones.

Most doctors say that a hysterectomy has no negative effect on your sexual responsiveness. I do not believe that the matter has been researched adequately enough to draw this conclusion. I have had several patients that are exceptions to the rule. One patient stopped having orgasms. Her orgasms were triggered by her husband thrusting against a spot deep in her vagina. As it turned out, her uterus had been tilted, so that the penis bumped it. When the uterus was removed, so was the familiar feeling, and she stopped responding. It was devastating to her sex life.

Hysterectomy usually has an emotional effect on the woman. Her reaction varies according to her personality and how she perceives the surgery. Some women are happily relieved to be free from menstruation or the pain they may have had from whatever disease process prompted the procedure, and glad to be without fear of pregnancy. If a woman sees hysterectomy as a symbol of aging, or the loss of her womanliness, however, it can cause varying degress of depression, and consequently, loss of interest in sex.

Usually overlooked is the psychological effect on the man. Most take the hysterectomy of their mates in stride. Some do not. One patient came for therapy because after her surgery, her husband refused to have sex with her again, although their sex life had been frequent and good quality before. He was a devout Catholic and felt that sex was not appropriate when there was no possibility of conceiving.

It is a good idea for a man and woman to discuss their feelings about hysterectomy prior to the surgery, and to see their physician together to ask all their questions and clear up any misconceptions that might exist.

Tilted Uterus

The most common cause of painful intercourse is constipation and one of the most common causes of constipation in women is a tilted uterus. The uterus rests against the bowels, and slows the transit time of body waste. Thus a woman can have a perfectly healthy uterus, but be constipated and somewhat uncomfortable with deep thrusting.

A tilted uterus is otherwise no problem, and doesn't require hysterectomy or resuspension surgery unless other medical problems coexist.

Vaginal Tightening Procedures

If you feel your vagina is too loose, it may be due to natural responsiveness.

The ballooning action of the vagina is responsible for something called "womb gas." When the inner two-thirds of the vagina balloons and the outer one-third constricts, air may be sucked into or out of the opening during thrusting and a woman may emit noise that sounds like passing gas. Sometimes after sex, when she sits up, relaxes, or takes a breath, the air that has been trapped in the inner ballooned part of the vagina is forced out, causing another embarrassing sound to occur. Many a woman, believing that the sounds she was emitting meant she was "too loose," has gone to her doctor for a tightening procedure to "fix" this problem. Surgical tightening is usually done on the outer third of the vagina, and cannot help or change what is a perfectly normal sexual response.

Womb gas is a sign of responsiveness and arousal, not looseness.

Some women have unnecessary tightening procedures done, but occasionally they are required. To find out, a doctor should measure you with more than his finger: Young's Dilators are useful for this purpose. Tightening procedures, when done, tighten the outlet only, and do not alter the looseness of the inner two-thirds of the vagina. Vaginal repairs are helpful if there has been muscle rupture, or tearing during delivery that was incompletely repaired at the time. Repairs are also done if the patient has such loose bladder support that she wets her pants when she coughs or sneezes or her vaginal-rectal wall bulges so she can't get feces out without pushing on the wall with her hand. Muscle tightening exercises (Kegel's exercises) can be done to increase the tone of the outer third of the vagina. There are instruments called perineometers to help you measure and exercise the strength of these muscles.

Genital Abuse

The things women do to their vaginas are sometimes hard to believe. One woman read somewhere that if she put an Alka Seltzer tablet on her clitoris, she would have an orgasm. She did not have an orgasm; instead, she had severe pain. The fizzing was supposed to be a turn-on, but it scratched up her tissues and made her feel miserable instead.

Another woman (after her husband told her that she was too loose) inserted alum into her vagina to shrink it. I don't even like to think about how she felt.

There is a physician who claims he is successfully making women orgasmic by improving on nature. He removes the clitoris from its normal location and reattaches it near the vaginal opening. In the process he disrupts the nerves. Be sure you clearly understand in advance just what procedure a physician plans to perform.

Clitoral Circumcision

Some doctors cut away the skin around your clitoris in a misdirected effort to make you have orgasms more easily. Don't have one done. It doesn't work; it makes matters worse by causing hypersensitivity; and it is an irreversible procedure.

Clitoridectomy

This is surgical removal of the clitoris. It is sometimes done for cancer of the vulva. In modern surgery the clitoris is spared unless that is where the cancer started. I have known patients whose doctors did not spell this out before surgery. The woman didn't specifically ask, and afterwards it was too late. Don't have the clitoris removed unless absolutely necessary, and only after a second or third opinion.

Clitoral Adhesionectomy

This procedure involves disrupting adhesions between the clitoris and the hood by inserting a blunt instrument, and breaking them apart. It is not generally harmful, but not generally useful either. Of the over 300 women studied at Master's and Johnson *who were able to be orgasmic*, 85 percent of them had clitoral adhesions. They are a normal occurrence.

Men's Pelvic Problems

Men are particularly fortunate. They do not get as many genital infections as women. Many of the infections they do get are asymptomatic (no symptoms), and rarely back up into the bladder to cause urinary tract problems. This makes sense because the distance from the skin surface to the bladder is much greater in the man than the woman, and germs have farther to travel. The infections they may get are rarely serious or life-threatening.

For example, as we mentioned in this chapter, men can harbor bacteria and yeast in their ejaculate without experiencing symptoms. It was formerly believed that a man couldn't be infected with gonorrhea unless he had "the drip." This is now known to be untrue. Some men carry the disease and do not show any symptoms.

Because men can harbor yeast, trichomonas, gonorrhea, hemophilus, and other infectious organisms, they are in a position of infecting their wives or lovers with unpleasant diseases without knowing it.

A couple who wanted badly to have another child underwent many medical tests. She had a history of numerous vaginal infections—trichomonas, yeast, and (unbeknownst to her) gonorrhea. When he got gonorrhea, she was treated with penicillin shots for "an infection that was going around the neighborhood," which was true, because so was he.

She developed PID (pelvic inflammatory disease, an inflammation of the tubes and uterus), which eventually subsided. She became pregnant, but due to scarring in her tubes, she had a tubal pregnancy. The tube ruptured and she almost bled to death before she could be gotten safely to surgery.

These problems would probably not have happened if they had had sex only with each other. The pattern of numerous different vaginal infections, pelvic inflammatory disease, ectopic pregnancy, and infertility suggests affairs.

The man, in this case, never intended to cause his wife these medical problems. He was as disappointed as she that they could have no more children. No doctor told either of them that his social behavior was affecting her medical health, although there had been many opportunities to do so. Therefore the progression of consequences could not be stopped.

Men who love their women, but who "fool around" on the side, can bring home problems that destroy health and sex. Herpes is another prime example of a venereally transmitted disease that can disrupt your sex life.

Local rashes, nonspecific urethritis (NSU)—an inflammation of the urethra—and prostatitis are the most common genital problems experienced by men.

All of these conditions can hang on stubbornly, and frequently become chronic. NSU and prostatitis can cause pain with urination and pain with ejaculation. Both can be brought on by having intercourse with a woman who has any of the vaginal infections described above.

Sporadic sexual activity—too much, too little, or too irregularly—has been held responsible for causing prostatitis.

Some cases of prostatitis and NSU are not treated *aggressively* enough. If the doctor has the person on antibiotics for two weeks, it is sometimes not long enough to eliminate the disease. If the medicine is helping, it should not be stopped until *all* the symptoms have disappeared—even if it takes months—or the inflammation will become chronic, and sometimes impossible to get rid of completely. Sometimes zinc tablets are added to the treatment to promote tissue healing, although their value has not been proven.

Masturbation is recommended, because the congested, inflamed prostate needs to be emptied regularly.

During my years as a doctor in the U.S. Navy, I treated many men—young and old—for this disorder. Prostatitis often surfaces among sailors. Their long sea voyages without regular sexual outlets make them more susceptible than the average civilian. Since masturbation was against regulations, I had to hand out signed "masturbation chits" for use if they were caught.

Peyronie's Disease

Peyronie's disease can be heartbreaking. It is a process which forms scar-like tissue inside the penis. This causes curvatures, and in some cases obstruction to the blood flow, causing impotence. The angulation can be severe enough to make intercourse impossible.

We don't know what causes this ailment, or how to prevent it. In some people it disappears by itself; in others it is progressive. Treatment—which can include ultrasound, surgery, or implants—is not always successful.

Trauma

Various other conditions affecting the pelvis—back injuries, spinal cord injuries, genital trauma, and surgeries—can complicate and impair your sex life. Among the surgeries, cancer surgery (especially for the bowel, prostate, and back) is the worst offender. Sexual complications can occur as a direct result of the surgery itself or as a result of complications associated with the surgery. Surgery can also cause impotence for *psychological* reasons. These problems require a careful medical and psychological workup. Trauma to the penis can damage the tissues sufficiently to cause permanent impotence. A sexually active sixty-two-year-old patient gave me the following history: He was visiting at the home of a new girlfriend. When he went to the bathroom, he was embarrassed at the noise he would make, so he got down on his knees to urinate. The toilet seat fell on his penis, causing intense pain. It was blue and swollen for several weeks and painful for months. After it healed, he was unable to become erect under any circumstances. He had ruptured the penile sheath (Buck's fascia) and thrombosed (clotted) strategic blood vessels.

Priapism

A permanent erection in a man who doesn't have an implant is called priapism. A man will sometimes get an erection and for some reason the blood flow from the penis is blocked and the erection will not drain. One cause can be a growth in the abdomen blocking blood flow out of the penis. A young man with this problem may have a cancerous gland or blood disease like lymphoma or a Hodgkin's disease. Fortunately, these two conditions are rare. Other diseases, such as sickle cell anemia, can also bring on this problem, but most of the time we can't really discover a cause.

The poor fellow usually comes into the emergency room about three days after he's gotten the erection. He was proud of it for the first two days; but now it's becoming painful and he wants to be rid of it. Sometimes unpleasant procedures such as inserting needles to drain the blood out are required. It may take a surgical operation to put new veins into the penis in order for blood flow to circulate again. If you develop an erection that does not subside, do not hesitate to call your doctor. Do not wait several days.

Prostate Surgery

Many men over the age of fifty have had prostate surgery. The most common type is done to correct a benign enlargement of the gland, using an instrument that is inserted through the penis. This operation does not cause impotence unless there are serious technical problems during the procedure. Sometimes the internal sphincter (muscle) to the bladder is damaged by the procedure, and the man may find that he doesn't ejaculate forward during orgasm. The semen goes backward instead of forward, ends up in the bladder, and is later expelled with the urine. This "backfiring," by the way, does not affect the sensation of orgasm—he can still enjoy it. Nor does it cause impotence.

Surgical procedures for cancer of the prostate usually cause impotence, but sometimes there are unpredictable, unexplainable exceptions.

I have had several male patients who had radical bladder,

prostate, or bowel surgeries performed. They "should" have become completely impotent but didn't.

One patient who had extensive bowel surgery for cancer of the rectum was told that he would be impotent for the rest of his life. Most men, after a sentence like that, wouldn't even experiment, but he did. He discovered that he could masturbate and get a pretty good erection (about 75 percent). However, he couldn't get erect with his wife, so he came to therapy. The inability to get equally erect with his wife was psychological, and psychotherapy was helpful.

Hints for Heart Patients and Those With Chronic Lung Disease

Doctors know more about how far you can run after a heart attack than about how much sex you can have. Which would you rather know?

If you are a cardiac patient, once you can walk one or two flights of stairs without symptoms, it should be safe to have sex. Men have been known to have intercourse in the hospital while recovering, but this is *not* wise.

Rest on your back. Let your partner do the physical work, and enjoy yourself. If you have angina, take a nitroglycerine pill before intercourse. Some even use their portable bedside oxygen during sex. Use your judgment and ingenuity.

A Popular Medical Syllogism

There are still many unanswered questions in medicine, and there is a popular medical syllogism which you should be aware of—and guard against. It goes like this:

1. In spite of many visits to the doctor, the problem is not cured.

2. Clearly, therefore, it does not exist.

3. Or it is somebody else's fault.

4. I cannot be at fault since I am a gynecologist (surgeon, neurologist, etc.).

5. Therefore it must be the patient's fault.

6. Send him (her) to a psychiatrist.

How many patients have been victims of this method? Have you ever felt the doctor was eyeing you suspiciously and not taking your physical complaints seriously?

A patient came to me several years ago. She had had no feeling in her vagina or clitoris since a back operation. She told her back surgeon and her neurologist but neither one reexamined her. They told her it was her attitude.

I saw her three years later. When I examined her, I found she had a permanent numbness in the "saddle block" distribution (the area that would touch the saddle if a woman was riding a horse).

She was able to learn to be orgasmic again, with breast stimulation. She never recovered sensation in the genitals, however. Her husband could enjoy intercourse with her, and so could she, as long as he also stimulated her breasts.

Many medical sexual problems cannot be found in textbooks. Ten years ago, medical science thought that less than 10 percent of all sexual problems were physical. Today, the guestimate is closer to 50 percent. I think this figure will go even higher as we learn more.

To solve medical sexual problems successfully requires a great deal of common sense, good judgment, and the cooperation of an open-minded, resourceful physician.

Dual Responsibility

There is a dual responsibility involved. You must spell out your problem in detail to your physician, just as you would do if you had gastrointestinal trouble; your physician must listen and ask pertinent questions.

Doctors learn how to ask embarrassing questions like "Do your stools float?" and, "What color are they?" We can certainly learn to ask our patients with some grace questions about masturbation and the nature of their sex lives.

You, the patient, must help by bringing the problem to your physician's attention, no matter how embarrassing it is to discuss.

The Team Effort

Many of the problems that seem beyond the scope of textbook medicine can be solved with a team effort. Far more can be accomplished today than you may think.

Painful intercourse should not be tolerated, and with a little knowledge, most of the genital diseases that interfere with sex can be prevented or caught early and treated effectively.

Hey Steve,

This is a good book. I'm a little ashamed, in reading this I've found & I've been believing a lot of myths (& me, a sociologist who's taken a class on the subject!)

(What's a threostat? @.40)

Note on p. 43, 5th sentence down from "expand beyond your genitals." I guess you're not so weird. (Note a line? Please note: nothing is said about jelly butters!

CHAPTER 14

New Advances in Sex Therapy (And Future Promises)

Medicine of the 1980s will provide an exciting new outlook on the treatment of sexual disorders.

The serious investigation of medicines to treat sexual difficulties is still in its infancy, but dramatic advances in the psychopharmacology of sex show great promise. In this decade drugs may emerge as the newest, fastest, and most effective means of treating sexual problems that once took many hours and sometimes years of therapy. These new techniques will give us the opportunity to correct previously untreatable problems. The use of specific drugs to treat sexual and emotional problems, combined with a clear and sensible understanding of the relationship between our mind and body will provide us with great versitility of treatment approaches.

Although psychiatry has used medicines to treat emotional problems for a long time, until recently we have not known how or why many of these drugs work. Highly skilled psychiatric professionals are using chemicals with delicate surgical precision to alter behavior and attitudes that are undesirable, emotionally crippling, or life-threatening.

We have learned that the presence or absence of certain substances in the body can influence your mood, prevent anxiety, cure depression, make you aggressive or docile, improve memory, affect appetite and combat anxiety. Prostaglandin inhibitors, a hormonelike medicine, are being used successfully to treat menstrual cramps. Aspirin can be used by heart attack victims as an anticoagulant to lessen the chance of a second seizure. Marijuana is being used to treat the nausea and vomiting caused by cancer chemotherapy. It is also being used to treat glaucoma. Heroin is helping to keep terminal cancer patients free from pain. Vasopressin, a hormone produced by the pituitary gland, stimulates memory in cases of amnesia, senility, and alcoholism. Cholecystokinin is a substance found lacking in obese mice and abundant in the brains of thin ones. Researchers are investigating the use of injections of cholecystokinin as a chemical cure for obesity, similar to treating diabetes with insulin. Dehydropiandrosterone (DHEA) is a steroid hormone that shows promise as a potential weapon against obesity, and perhaps the aging process. As medical research continues to make progress, substances to retard aging and to increase sexual desire are closer to becoming a reality.

The Psychopharmacology of Sex Simplified

A few years ago, an obscure medical journal reported that L-Dopa, a medicine used for treatment of Parkinsonism in older men, had a disturbing side effect: it caused septuagenarians to climb the bedrails in nursing homes in search of women—any women. The effect on their libido was so pronounced that the drug became a real nuisance to the nurses charged with their care. The popular press picked up this item and poked a little fun at it. Researchers are currently investigating the value of this drug in treating men and women with low sex drives.

Testosterone is the only known drug that can be considered a true aphrodisiac—*in women,* that is. In low doses, it causes a marked increase in sexual arousal. Unfortunately, women exposed to it for any significant length of time grow beards, and get hair on their chests. Their voices get lower by about an octave and they get bold and bald.

The tranquilizers Mellaril and thioridazine have been in use for many years, and their benefits are well known to most psychiatrists. One of their adverse side effects, however, is that males taking the drugs find it difficult or impossible to ejaculate. The implications here are interesting: while their effect on ejaculation might be a drawback to men without sexual difficulty, those who experience premature ejaculation might find their use highly desirable.

A specific group of drugs imitates the effects of adrenalin; another group of drugs blocks those effects. Among the medicines that block adrenalin is Propranolol (a heart medicine), which is used by musicians, actors, and public speakers to counteract stage fright. Propranolol prevents the cold chills, trembling, rapid heart rate, sweating, and other symptoms by blocking the action of adrenalin on blood vessels and nerves. Such a drug could possibly stop the effect of fear on the erection, thus sustaining the erection in a stressed situation.

Because these blocking drugs are powerful and affect other parts of your body, particularly your heart, they are not innocuous, and must be investigated with caution. In their most typical use, for the treatment of heart disease, such drugs are administered in strong doses, and have been blamed for causing impotence. Their use is not uncomplicated and their value will depend on the extent of their side effects as well as their direct action on sexual function.

For those sexual dysfunctions that are psychological in origin, how can drugs be of much value?

Psychological impotence actually results from a chemical released within our body, one triggered by fear (remember the adrenalin reflex). As noted above, one group of drugs imitates the effects of adrenalin, while another blocks the effects of adrenalin. A drug that prevents the action of adrenalin on blood vessels and nerves could well interfere with the effect of fear on the erection. By preventing the blood vessels from constricting, the erection can be sustained during stress. Since adrenalin also stimulates ejaculation, you can see that a drug that could block the adrenalin effect also has the potential of slowing or inhibiting ejaculation, and could be used for the treatment of premature ejaculation.

Pheromones—Sexual Perfume?

Pheromones are naturally occurring substances that animals secrete. Their odor causes specific behavior. Wolves and dogs mark their territory with the pheromones in their urine. Other wolves smell the pheromone and know that they are trespassing. Female dogs in heat emit a sexual pheromone that sends all the male dogs in the neighborhood into a sexual frenzy.

Researchers have discovered and duplicated a sexual pheromone in cockroaches. "Why would they do that?" you ask. The synthetic pheromone is used as a pesticide. It is sprayed in a spot. When the male cockroaches attracted to it congregate in one area, they are exterminated. A practical roach approach to birth control, perhaps, but not suitable for humans.

Studies of sexual pheromones in humans are currently underway. The International Federation of Flavors and Fragrances would like to bottle it, give it a French name, and control the world. Human sexual pheromones, once they are identified and synthesized, will be THE aphrodisiac.

Jovan, Inc. has introduced Andron, a perfume containing synthetically produced quantities of alpha androstenol. The scent is actually derived from androstenone, a pheromone or "chemical messenger" of the boar.

A recent survey at Georgetown University's Taste and Smell Clinic showed that 25 percent of people with smell disorders lose interest in sex. Independent research in other centers supports the concept that olfactory cues may play a more significant role in our sexual behavior than we realize.

Soviet physicians are also experimenting with pheromone therapy. They hope to demonstrate that certain chemical combinations sprayed into the environment (such as hospital rooms) can soothe anxiety, ease stress, and even induce hypnosis and sleep. The use of subtle odors as hidden persuaders has perhaps also occurred to them.

Copulins

Copulins are fatty acids found in the vaginal secretions of female rhesus monkeys. They powerfully stimulate the sexual interest of the male rhesus monkey. They are also present in human females. Unfortunately, human experiments have been inconclusive.

Mixed Signals

Another study done on rhesus monkeys found that if you take a tampon from a menstruating female and smear it on the genitals of a nonmenstruating rhesus female, it arouses the male rhesus even more than when she is in natural estrus (menstruation).

Odors related to human menstruation have not been studied extensively. Horseback riders know that a stallion will react to a menstruating woman the same way he reacts to a mare in heat. As a result, during seven days out of each month it is almost impossible for a woman to ride a stallion. It is also not wise to go swimming in shark-filled waters.

There are other indications that certain animals respond to the scents of a menstruating woman. Two girls were attacked and killed by grizzly bears in the wilderness of Montana. Both were having their periods. A seventy-five-year-old woman from Oklahoma told me that none of the women go into the hills during their period because of the risk of attack by wolves, hogs, and other animals that do not disturb them during the rest of their cycle. This information is not generally known among women. It is not widely known among professionals either. Yet the knowledge could be lifesaving under certain circumstances in the wilderness. Think about your twelve-year-old daughter on her first Girl Scout camping trip in the Sierras.

A recent letter in the *Medical Journal of Australia* stated that female lion tamers are at a disadvantage: apparently lions are more apt to attack a woman who is menstruating. A prospective female lion tamer, aware of these occupational hazards, asked her physician to remove her uterus. Her doctor concluded that this was a "rare but genuine indication for hysterectomy."

When the biological chemical signals sometimes unexpectedly cross species barriers, it can be dangerous.

Is There Chemistry?

Another study was done that was also most revealing. Three odors were put in containers and men were asked to smell them.

One of the odors consisted of female vaginal secretions, although the men were not aware of this. The physiological responses of the men were measured during the experiment: skin temperature, pulse rate, heartbeat, etc., and they were then asked to describe the odors. They described the vaginal secretions as smelling fishy, but they gave no indication that they were aroused. However, of all the preparations they were exposed to, only the vaginal odors caused increased blood pressure, heart rate, and skin temperature. The body's physiological responses to vaginal odors were too subtle for the men to detect subjectively, but something happened—a response that was recordable on machinery.

Love at First Sight

These studies suggest that we have a lot to learn. There may be something to what you hear described so often as "love at first sight." You see someone, you get near them, and respond to a dynamic physical attraction. Is it pheromones? I don't know. Something chemical is happening. We even use the term "chemical attraction." It is fascinating to think about, and we hope to have many answers in the next decade or two.

A psychiatrist at New York State Psychiatric Institute says that phenylethylamine—an amphetamine-like mood-altering drug found in the brain—is the cause of the giddiness and happiness associated with romance. Since chocolate contains phenylethylamine, candy bars could come in handy when starting or ending a love affair.

Substances that alter sex drive have been searched for eagerly throughout history. A not-so-distant example: cold breakfast cereals were originally produced to dampen the human sex drive. John Harvey Kellogg said in 1906 that children who ate his cereal instead of bacon and eggs wouldn't fall prey to the sin of "self-pollution," a euphemism for masturbation.

Pheromones are more than cereal, and even more than sexual messages. They are orders. An insect has no choice but to obey its chemistry. Many men and women passionately in love have felt that they were the helpless "victim" of some outside force, too.

However, in a society that has now deodorized almost everything in sight, there is doubt about the degree of our sensitivity to perceive pheromones even if they do indeed exist. Is it possible that our social conditioning and programming has made them irrelevant, or diluted our reactions so significantly that what would have caused an orgy centuries ago, now barely gets a wink?

What will be the consequences if these long-distance hormones are found? To what use will they be put? Speculations abound and have been the focus of many science-fiction articles. The possibilities challenge the imagination: arousal dysfunctions might easily be treated with this chemical; love potions could be brewed and tried on desirable mates or partners whose ardor has cooled.

Grafenberg's Spot

The Grafenberg spot and female ejaculation have been discussed at some length in Chapter 7. The anatomy and histology of Graffenberg's spot is being studied by the Crenshaw Clinic, Dr. Kurt Bernischke, Dr. Purvis Martin, and others. Research in these areas should be available in the immediate future—and may have a profound influence on the diagnosis, classification, and treatment of women's orgasmic problems.

A New Form of Testosterone

Recently, two manifestations of the hormone testosterone have been discovered: a free form and a bound form. Until now, the measurement of the total testosterone has not correlated well with sex drive: men with high levels could have low sex drives and vice versa. Other hormone systems, such as the thyroid, contain both a free and bound form. The bound form is attached to a protein and is metabolically inactive, which means it is basically dormant. The free form that circulates in the blood stream is active. If testosterone operates in the same way, a man could have a very high level of testosterone with no effect at all on libido or erection if it is in the inactive bound form. Approximately 10 percent of the testosterone is in the unbound form. (In females over 95 percent of the circulating testosterone is bound to proteins.) On the other hand, one could have a low total testosterone level, but if 50 percent of it is in the free form, it could produce a strong sexual function despite the low total value. These interpretations are speculative, but current research promises to increase our understanding of these complex hormonal relationships.

Hyperprolactinemia—a Newly Discovered Cause of Impotence

Masters and Johnson recently identified that hyperprolactinemia causes loss of libido and impotence in men. It is a rare disorder, but can be determined by blood studies of testosterone, prolactin, FSH (follicle-stimulating hormone) and LH (luteinizing hormone). This problem can be successfully treated surgically or chemically if diagnosed early.

Have We Discovered the Control Center?

A compound known as LHRH (luteinizing-hormone-releasing hormone) may be a key to human sexual activity. It affects both the body and the mind. It is the chemical signal that controls the sex hormones, and is one of the newly discovered groups of chemicals that may be intimately involved in memory, emotion, and the perception of pain. Its possible application in the treatment of impotence is also being explored. LHRH holds promise of being the first unisex birth control drug—a contraceptive that would work in both men and women.

LHRH is concentrated in parts of the rat brain that govern sexual behavior. When LHRH-derived drugs act on these rodents' brains they send the animals into a mating pattern.

The Chinese have used LHRH analogs to encourage carp to spawn and have used them experimentally in breeding pandas. There are no comparable human experiments, but its use in the treatment of low sex drive in the human is also being researched.

Bromocryptine is a synthetic agent derived from a fungus. A few years ago a group of Italian researchers reported that the drug restored desire and potency to men and women who had lost the urge, and even to some who had "never had an erotic feeling in their entire lives.'' Bromocryptine inhibits the production of prolactin, a chemical associated with lower levels of sex hormones; it is currently one of the methods being used to treat hyperprolactinemia. It may also influence dopamine and serotonin metabolism, two substances in the brain that regulate mood, and may turn out to be one of the most promising drugs in the treatment of sexual disorders of the future. However, the human sex drive is complex, and no single chemical is likely to be the complete answer.

The Nocturnal Penile Tumescence Monitor and the Inflatable Penile Prosthesis

The nocturnal penile tumescence monitor (Peter Meter) and the inflatable penile prosthesis (Bionic Penis) discussed in Chapter 12, are among the most important advances in the last decade in the diagnosis and treatment of impotence. A penile doppler (blood flow indicator) tests the blood flow to the penis, and X-ray studies examine the vessels of the penis for disease and mechanical blockage. And just as there are bypass operations for the heart, there are bypass operations for the penis: a blood vessel is transplanted from another area of the body to the penis to bypass the blockage that is preventing erection. This bypass procedure, however, does not have a high success rate, and needs to be perfected.

Electroejaculation

An even newer and more intricate approach to the treatment of physiological impotence is electroejaculation. This method is currently only available to patients in a research setting, and will need extensive modifications before it can be useful as a treatment method.

Electroejaculation has been done in animals for many years. For example, it is a routine way of fertilizing a large number of cows from one prize bull while preventing any risk of injury to the bull. Experts in the field can now electroejaculate creatures in many species—from a gorilla to an armadillo. Again, you might ask, and understandably so, "Why would anyone want to do that?"

Zoos are quite interested in breeding their animals successfully, especially the rare or expensive ones, but they want to protect their valuable display of animals from injuries—especially those that can occur during natural mating. Many animals who have been raised in captivity do not even know how to mate, and electroejaculation followed by artificial insemination has been a frequent solution to this dilemma.

Pete and Gladys

In the early months of my practice, I was asked to consult on two rather unusual patients: Pete and Gladys, a pair of spectacled bears at the San Diego Zoo, were experiencing a sexual problem. I normally don't make house calls, but in this case decided against having them come to the clinic. I was told that these bears (from the Peruvian Andes) are an endangered species. Laws governing the importation of animals prevented the zoo from acquiring more of these rare creatures and officials there were very anxious to have this pair breed.

Gladys had given birth once, but—not having taken any motherhood training—she ate her babies before anyone could stop her. Pete had developed a nervous problem called alopecia ariata, as a result of which he had lost all of his hair. The zoo didn't think he made a very good display bear, bald, and, eventually took him off exhibit until his hair grew back. Clearly, there were enough deep-rooted problems to make any psychoanalyst shudder with delight.

However, the event that prompted the zoo committee to consult a sex therapist was Pete's peculiar behavior. Instead of mounting Gladys to relieve his sexual tension, he would sit in a corner in full view of zoo patrons and suck on his penis—while purring with a noise that imitated the sound of a Mack truck. He became known as the X-rated bear. Bus drivers would not stop before his cage, and old ladies would stand there for hours shaking their heads disapprovingly.

Pete, this glaring source of embarrassment, underwent many studies to determine the cause of his disinterest in Gladys.

Finally, electroejaculation was ordered, so his sperm could be examined to discover if he was in fact fertile. During that episode, sex therapist and expert in electroejaculation met.

Pete and Gladys, however, were not impressed. Gladys never had children. In bear years, she turned out to be too old to have more babies. She contented herself by swopping Pete with all of her might whenever she noticed him sitting in the corner enjoying himself.

A research study on humans was a natural outgrowth of this bear case. No one had yet succeeded in electroejaculating human beings. The research was performed at the Crenshaw Clinic, in conjunction with Yerkes Primate Center and Emory University. The electroejaculation study was funded by the National Institute of Mental Health and completed two years later. The technique developed was successful.

An electrode is inserted into the rectum. Then current is applied until an erection and ejaculation occur. At present, the voltage necessary is higher than can be comfortably tolerated by a normal man. Consequently, the procedure has only been successful in spinal injury patients who are numb below the waist. Portable units for home use may someday be available by prescription to spinal injury patients who could benefit from them.

An Overview

Sexual devices, toys, and gadgets are developing with amazing speed. We already have equipment to measure nocturnal erections and penile blood flow. Surgical procedures can now correct impotence. The inflatable implant can restore erections to men who were previously incapable, and penile bypass procedures are being refined.

The adrenalin reflex has increased our understanding and improved the treatment of psychological impotence.

Research is underway on a new form of testosterone. Various drugs show promise in the treatment of premature ejaculation, ejaculatory incompetence, erective difficulties, and orgasmic problems.

The search for the ultimate aphrodisiac is seriously underway with pheromones, copulins, and other substances competing for that position.

We may soon prove that women do, indeed, ejaculate. Graffenberg's spot could turn out to be a significant finding. Whether it exists or not, I am sure that couples all over the world will enjoy looking for it. Electroejaculation devices for men and women may someday replace the vibrator in the bedside table. We already have the ability to change one sex into another, and can successfully raise test tube babies.

Research in these areas has been building momentum for decades. The results are just starting to surface. I believe that the 1980s will see sexual medicine emerge as one of the most exciting new disciplines of the century.

From Mechanics to Biochemistry

However, techniques and devices are not enough. An implant can't bridge emotional rifts. An orgasm can't save a shaky marriage. Our emphasis is still too often on performance instead of feelings. Without tenderness, love, caring, intimacy, and support, sex suffers, no matter how fine your plumbing is.

New discoveries about the biochemistry of emotions have shaken the foundations of medicine, philosophy, and psychology.

Emotional and psychological patterns among men and women have been attributed to environmental factors, but now the emphasis is changing. Data from the right/left hemisphere brain studies (described in Chapter 5) and new theories proposed by sociobiology are challenging many of our trusted preconceived notions.

Anke Ehrhardt, Patricia Goldman, Sarah Blaffer Hrdy, Corinne Hutt, Julianne Imperato-McGinley are but a few distinguished women scientists who devote their lives to the study of the brain, hormones, or behavior, both human and animal. They have all concluded that sex differences in behavior between men and women are at least, in part, biological.

In spite of studies in children and adults demonstrating sex-linked differences (now given greater credibility by the identification of brain differences), political views make it difficult to interpret this information without bias. All the data isn't in yet. It is too early for sweeping conclusions. The information surfacing is nonetheless fascinating, and will lead to considerable controversy.

Hormones and Behavior

It is thought that the hypothalamus (a tiny section in the brain) governs much of our human behavior, including our moods, our sex drives, and our emotions. Modern methods of treating depression successfully with mood elevators confirms this biochemical link. It is even suspected that depression is a genetic marker in residence on chromosome number 6.

Some medicines used in treating disease eliminate sex drive (like certain cardiac drugs) or increase it (like L-Dopa). Although we do not yet understand the mechanisms of their action, it is reasonable to assume that we will eventually be able to treat sexual desire problems, impotence, premature ejaculation, and orgasmic problems with drugs too—even those now considered to be psychological problems. Some avant-garde researchers consider psychology and biochemistry to be the same thing.

A close look at male and female hormones gives us fascinating information about ourselves. These substances determine how we look. Is it so far-fetched to consider that they also affect how we feel?

If you give a man estrogen, his breasts enlarge and he redistributes his tissues—sometimes so successfully that he cannot be distinguished from a woman (as female impersonators in nightclub acts demonstrate); it affects his emotions by making him docile, more passive, and reducing his sex drive.

Not surprisingly, testosterone causes a woman's body to become more like a man's: her voice deepens, her muscles bulk, and she grows more body hair. It affects her emotions too. She becomes more aggressive, and her sex drive increases.

Songbirds and Japanese Fighting Fish

Other findings suggest that biochemistry is responsible for some of the behavioral and emotional differences between men and women. Rapists, exhibitionists, and perpetrators of violent crime have higher testosterone levels than normal men. Japanese fighting fish are even more aggressive than normal if they happen to have double male chromosomes. Men confined in crowded quarters (such as military barracks) have lower testosterone than when living separately. Perhaps it is because they must reduce aggression in order to survive.

If you give female canaries testosterone, they will start to sing (usually only the male does).

In the Great Tit, by and large, song is produced by males and not the females. A female Great Tit has been observed in full song defending the territory when her mate was sick for a few days. When he recovered, she stopped singing. These exceptions suggest that the female of the species may be capable of many other things, including singing, but often doesn't manifest a talent unless necessary.

Premenstrual Tension—Fact or Fiction?

Women in harems and students in dormitories adjust to the same menstrual cycle. That is why sultans kept a number of women in a separate tent. Imagine two hundred premenstrual women under the same roof.

More crimes are committed by women during their premenstrual phase, according to some studies. Recently, two women in Britain involved in separate murders, had their sentences reduced: premenstrual tension was given as the mitigating reason. They were judged to have "diminished responsibility." Extreme? Perhaps, perhaps not.

Incidentally, premenstrual women are experiencing estrogen withdrawal (their levels are low), which means that the testosterone they normally have in their system is freer to influence them—and indeed many women report that their sex drives are considerably higher at that time.

When I was still in medical school, premenstrual tension was considered a condition of women whose misguided mothers called menstruation "the curse." I concluded that if premenstrual tension was all the result of how we were raised, our closest relatives—the primates—would not have it; so I investigated by contacting numerous zoos and primate centers.

Premenstrually (prior to estrus) the rhesus monkey gains up to five pounds, which are lost as estrus begins. Usually calm and agreeable, they become irritable and aggressive. They bite their mate and chatter at their offspring. Cage handlers and keepers can tell when estrus is approaching without checking the charts, because these normally cooperative animals cannot be handled safely at that time without risk of biting or other mischief.

Since mother rhesus did not poison her offsprings' minds, these behavior changes were clearly physiologically programmed.

The depression, weight gain, water retention, irritability, aggressiveness, hysteria, pelvic heaviness, abdominal cramping, backache, and lethargy of premenstrual tension in women are all too real, and sometimes trigger severe arguments, violence, divorce, and even suicide.

A woman who is well informed anticipates her emotional and physical condition and corrects for it in the same way she would handle hypoglycemia or a mild cold.

All women do not have premenstrual tension, but we do not know what percent of women experience the syndrome.

Menopause has also gained respect as a medical rather than hysterical condition, and for the first time serious study is being directed to investigate if and how men's emotions vary cyclically.

What Does It All Mean?

The wealth of new information that is surfacing raises as many questions as it answers.

A sexual dysfunction is a matter of opinion, determined by a society and the professionals in it. The definitions change with time and new attitudes.

By today's standards, our specific sexual problems are: the inability to be orgasmic, painful intercourse, an unconsummated marriage, impotence, premature ejaculation, ejaculatory incompetence, sexual aversion, and other arousal dysfunctions.

Believe it or not, some people can have a wonderful sex life in spite of these "technical problems." It is then a matter of defining the problem and finding the best solution.

On a deeper level is consideration of the relationship. No

matter how diligently you work to fix someone's plumbing, if the person does not want to plumb with someone else the result is nil. If two people don't like each other, can't communicate, and have festering resentments, sex alone can't make things all right. As a matter of fact, under these conditions, sex usually won't work at all even if both people are perfectly normal physically.

Sex can improve a good marriage and help a faltering one— but it can't rescue a disaster.

You cannot treat sex in a vacuum; it must be considered in the context of the whole person. If that person is in a relationship, that, too, must be carefully considered. Individuals function differently in different settings under different circumstances. However, their basic nature will follow them: with one man or woman they may function better than with another, but sooner or later underlying problems will surface. Occasionally, a person with a problem finds another individual with a compatible problem. The result can be that their lives together are far better than they could ever be separately.

Bear in mind that while many things are biologically possible and are there should you want them—all of it is by no means necessary for a well-adjusted and superlative sex life. People's standards and expectations are constantly changing; so instead of trying to keep up with every new idea, find out what pleases you the most and stick with it.

Sexually, men and women often have distinctly different needs, which cannot be adequately satisfied by the manners and attitudes we have been taught up to now. A more functional sexual etiquette that takes feelings into account, combined with basic common sense, will take sex beyond the "sexual revolution" and into our everyday lives. It can serve to strengthen the bonds between men and women and enable us to deal more successfully with the challenges involved in living and loving together.

CHAPTER 15

Self-Evaluation Questionnaires

Who Has the Problem, What Would You Call It, and What Can Be Done About It?

This chapter is designed to help you evaluate your own sex life; to determine whether you are developing a problem; to find out if you already have one and just don't know it; and to help you to decide what to do about it.

If you think you have a problem, that is a problem in itself. The self-assessment questionnaires will help you decide whether or not you actually do.

If you are impotent, the test will take you through a logical sequence of questions that will pinpoint the cause as physical or psychological.

If you are a woman who is unable to reach orgasm, or takes too long to do so, the questionnaire will help you identify the reason. If you have pain with intercourse, even if you have been told over and over again that there is nothing physically wrong, you will be in a position to find the cause and better guide your physician in making a diagnosis.

If you are a premature ejaculator, you will understand the degree and severity of your problem and be able to pursue appropriate avenues for change.

If you have a problem, you will know what it is, or you will know what further steps must be taken for a definitive diagnosis; and you will be knowledgeable enough to select among the forms of treatment available.

Most of us understand a cold. We know what to do when we get one (come in out of the cold, lots of chicken soup, etc.). We also know the warning signs of a more serious condition developing—persistent cough, wheezing, chest pain—and we know when to get help.

We have no such perspective on sex. We are unable to distinguish between mild and severe symptoms. We don't know when to come in out of the (sexual) cold and get medical attention. If we knew as little about colds as we do about sex, we would have trouble taking care of ourselves: we wouldn't know to take decongestants, be alert for ear infections in babies, or know the symptoms of bronchitis and pneumonia.

With this fundamental, but sophisticated information, you can apply native intelligence to recognize a sexual problem in the early stages and probably solve it yourself.

At a cocktail party the other night, a woman said to me, "I am so relieved to see sexual problems being written about. I read an article in an airline magazine that says impotence happens at one time or another to every man, and not to worry about it. My husband's eighteen-year-old son is impotent and is behaving like it is the end of the world. We told him not to worry."

Impotence in an eighteen-year-old boy is not the end of the world; nor is it something, however, to ignore with the nonchalance with which we advise someone about a stuffy nose, "It's just a cold, it will pass." It is more like a bronchitis that could progress into pneumonia. Proper treatment can stop it. Neglect might cause it to become acute or chronic.

Use these questionnaires as guides, not absolutes. The specific logical sequence of questions will help you use your common sense and the information in this book to assess your own sexuality.

Self-Evaluation Questionnaires for Men

SEXUAL SELF-ASSESSMENT

1. Do you ever have difficulty getting or sustaining an erection?
2. Do you ever lose erections (other than after ejaculating)?
3. Do you have any difficulty with ejaculation?
   a. Are you unable to ejaculate under certain circumstances?
   b. Do you feel that you ejaculate too quickly?

---

4. Have you ever ejaculated without direct penile manipulation?
5. Do you ever have pain with intercourse?
6. Have you experienced ejaculation through a flaccid (soft) penis?
7. As a rule, do you desire sex more often or less often than your partner?
8. Does your partner have any problems with arousal, orgasm, or lubrication?
9. Has there been any decrease in your:
   a. sex drive?
   b. frequency of intercourse?
   c. frequency or firmness of morning erection?
10. Do you have any difficulty becoming erect or orgasmic during masturbation?

If you have answered yes to *any* of the above questions, you *may* have a sexual problem and should read the interpretation which follows.

Interpretation

A positive response to any one of the questions does not mean that something is wrong with you. It merely suggests that further evaluation is warranted. If you answered yes to three or more of these questions, you probably already have such a problem.

If you answered yes to **1** and **2,** you are experiencing erective insecurity. This state usually leads to impotence. If, in addition, you have answered yes to **6, 9c,** and **10,** you are probably already impotent, and the problem may be severe.

If you said yes to **3b,** you are either a premature ejaculator, or predisposing yourself to impotence. If **4** is also true for you, you are probably a relatively severe premature ejaculator.

If **7, 9a,** and **9b** are true, you are on your way to becoming sexually aversive.

If **9a, 9b,** and **9c** are true, impotence of a physical nature may be developing.

Reviewing the implications of each of these questions individually will help you understand their importance and the rationale behind them.

1: Do you ever have difficulty getting or sustaining an erection?

If you have difficulty obtaining or sustaining an erection, you are probably entering each sexual encounter with some degree of apprehension (especially with a new partner). This state of mind makes you susceptible to the adrenalin reflex (Chapter 12), which causes the inability to get an erection.

2: Do you lose erections (other than after ejaculating)?

If, after becoming involved, you lose erections, it is likely that distractions, stress, pressure, or fears of performance are affecting you in some way—or you have turned sex into work. However, keep in mind that it is perfectly normal not to be erect if you are not aroused.

3: Do you have any difficulty with ejaculation?

    a. Are you unable to ejaculate under certain circumstances?

If you are unable to ejaculate occasionally, there is usually nothing wrong. However, if you are fairly *consistently* unable to ejaculate with intercourse, or with one woman but not another, or with oral sex but not with intercourse, etc., there is a psychological problem and you may be developing ejaculatory incompetence, which is the inability to ejaculate.

    b. Do you feel that you ejaculate too quickly?

If you *believe* you ejaculate too quickly, even if you actually last longer than average, the anxiety itself eventually can cause impotence. If you are indeed ejaculating rapidly and don't correct the problem, that too usually leads to impotence. The distress you experience and your efforts to think of other things in order to last longer, take the pleasure out of sex. When you are finally successful in tuning out, so does your erection.

4: Have you ever ejaculated without direct penile manipulation?

If you have ejaculated spontaneously (with the exception of nocturnal emissions), under stress, or climbing a rope, you are probably a severe premature ejaculator. You may barely be able to penetrate or thrust before it is over. This problem will not go away by itself. No matter how hard you try to discipline your mind, unless you get some professional help you will only succeed in making yourself impotent or aversive. Talk therapy alone is not adequate. The squeeze technique, properly prescribed, is essential.

5: Do you ever have pain with intercourse?

If you have persistent pain with intercourse or with ejaculation that does not respond to treatment, you are headed toward impotence. It doesn't matter if it only hurts for a little while; pain and sexual arousal in the normal male cannot coexist.

6: Have you experienced ejaculation through a flaccid (soft) penis?

Ejaculation and erection can occur independently. A man can be erect and not ejaculate, or be able to ejaculate without being erect. Ejaculation through a nonerect penis can be a sign of advanced impotence.

7: As a rule do you desire sex more often or less often than your partner?

The important phrase here is *as a rule*. Most people have different sexual appetites. If, however, you always want sex more (or less) than your partner, sexual stresses will invariably develop. They will become progressively worse if they are unattended, usually resulting in sexual aversion for one or both of you.

8: Does your partner have any problems with arousal, orgasm, or lubrication?

If your partner has a sexual problem of any kind that persists for months or years, it is quite probably that you will become sexually aversive, or even impotent. If you care for her, seeing her dissatisfaction and frustration can't help but affect you. You may have tried to help in every way you can, and turned sex into a big chore for yourself. This, too, can lead to impotence.

9: Has there been any decrease in your . . .
    a. sex drive?

If your sex drive has decreased gradually over the years, a problem is sneaking up on you. Take another look at your relationship and attack the problem before it gets too advanced.

    b. frequency of intercourse?

If frequency has decreased, but your sex drive hasn't, there is a problem brewing within either you or your partner. If both your drive and frequency are low, sexual aversion is already advanced.

c. frequency or firmness of morning erection?

If the firmness or the frequency of your morning erection is diminishing, some serious problems could be developing. If you are impotent and these changes occur, it could be a physical problem. Don't put off finding out what's wrong.

10: Do you have any difficulty becoming erect or orgasmic during masturbation?

No matter how impotent you think you are, it is all in your mind if you can still masturbate without difficulty. If you get a good erection with masturbation, and can ejaculate as easily as you used to, you are physiologically functioning just fine. The adrenalin reflex is having its way with you when you are with your mate.

If you have problems with masturbation as well as with a partner, the problem could be either psychological, or physical or both.

IMPOTENCE

The following questions will help you determine the causes of your impotence. When you have completed this questionnaire, go on to read the interpretation of your responses.

Erections are graded on a scale of 0–10. 0 is a completely flaccid (or limp) penis. 10 is a completely erect penis. Half an erection would be graded as a 5.

1. When was the very first time in your life that you can remember losing an erection, or not getting one, at a time that you thought was inappropriate? Include those times that you were drunk or tired.
2. When was the very next time that you lost an erection after gaining one, or could not get an erection at all?
3. When did the loss of erections equal the number of successful intercourse opportunities? In other words, when did you lose erections 50 percent of the time?
4. When was the last time that you had intercourse?
5. How frequently now are you attempting intercourse? How

frequently do you succeed? How frequently do you think about intercourse?

6. Have you ever ejaculated (had an orgasm) through a flaccid or limp penis?

7. What is the best grade erection you have had under any circumstances during recent months? What were the circumstances?

8. Grade your erections on a scale of 0–10.
  a. morning erections?
  b. nighttime erections?
  c. erections with masturbation?
  d. erections with partner stimulation (manual)?
  e. erections with partner stimulation (oral)?
      (1) with her mouth on your genitals?
      (2) with your mouth on her genitals?
  f. erections with fantasy only?
  g. erections with intercourse?
  h. erections with extramarital sex?
  i. erections with prostitute experience?
  j. other?

9. When do you most typically lose erections?

10. How frequently do you masturbate?

11. Do you fantasize during masturbation? During intercourse?

12. What is the state of your general health?

13. What medications are you taking?

14. Do you smoke tobacco? How many packs/day?

15. Do you drink alcohol? How many ounces/day?

16. What contraceptive method are you using?

17. Grade your relationship or marriage on a 0–10 scale. *(0 signifies a very unhappy marriage and 10 signifies a very happy one.)*

18. Do you avoid dating because of sexual difficulties?

Interpretation

1: When was the very first time in your life that you can remember losing an erection, or not getting one, at a time that you thought was inappropriate?

That will tell you when the problem first began, and what triggered it originally. Was it alcohol? The pressure of an unfamiliar situation? A new woman you were trying to please? Fatigue?

2: When was the very next time that you lost an erection after gaining one, or could not get an erection at all?

The time passed between your first episode and your second could be a few hours or many years. This information will give you a gauge of the progressive severity of the erective insecurity.

3: When did the loss of erections equal the number of successful intercourse opportunities?

When you are unable to have intercourse 50 percent of the attempts, you are "technically" impotent by the current definition. In general, at that point the erective insecurity is severe enough to be considered a sexual dysfunction. Thus, most men are concerned about their sexual potency long before they are unable to function half the time.

4: When was the last time that you had intercourse?

This tells you when the problem got so severe you couldn't function at all.

Men often come in for help thinking of a long-standing problem as a recent one because they don't register it as a "real problem" until they are completely unable to function.

Fill in the blanks of this sentence, and you may surprise yourself with the perspective you develop.

The first time I couldn't get an erection I was———years old. I began losing erections———(days, months, years) later. By the time I was———I couldn't have intercourse half the time I tried. Then when I was———I couldn't have intercourse at all. That was———(weeks, months, years) ago.

A common picture would be: The first time I ever had a problem was when I was seventeen—which was the first time I tried. I couldn't get erect at all. I didn't date again for two years—I was too embarrassed. With the next girl, I had a little trouble in the beginning, but it all worked out. I didn't have any more problems until I was thirty-five. After ten years of marriage, I started losing a few erections now and then, but didn't worry about it. By the time I was forty, though, it was happening about half the time. Now I can't get erect at all. I am fifty-eight and haven't had intercourse for eleven years.

This man may date the problem since age forty-seven, when he stopped being able to have intercourse, but the seeds were present at age seventeen. Use of therapy, or a book like this, at a young age would prevent the development of impotence altogether.

5: How frequently now are you attempting intercourse? How frequently do you succeed? How frequently do you think about intercourse?

Question 5 is particularly important.

If you are still trying, even if you never succeed, sexual aversion probably hasn't set in yet. If you are not trying, it suggests that you are resigned to impotence. Sexual aversion has set in, and you are depressed to some degree whether you recognize it or not. If you think about sex often, when unable to have it, you may be severely depressed. Some impotent men say, "Even though I don't miss sex, I think about it all the time—the fact that I can't have it if I wanted to bothers me, and I don't feel like a complete man. It seems like everyone knows— like they can tell."

6: Have you ever ejaculated (had an orgasm) through a flaccid or limp penis?

If the answer is yes, you can still be orgasmic, although the erection is no longer there. It usually requires vigorous stimulation to ejaculate without an erection, and it takes longer. Nonetheless, your neurological and physiological mechanism for orgasm is intact. Since most men assume one isn't possible without the other, they don't even try. *If* the cause is medical, you are a good candidate for an implant, which can provide an erection, but not the ability to ejaculate if it isn't already there.

7: What is the best grade erection you have had under any circumstances during recent months? What were the circumstances?

If you have had a grade 10 erection under any circumstances, we know that you are biologically intact. If there were structural or mechanical damage such as blocked penile vessels from arteriosclerosis, you would never have a grade 10 under any circumstances.

A grade 10 erection means the tissue is healthy and the hydrodynamic mechanism responsible for filling the penis works properly.

8: Grade your erections on a scale of 0–10.
   a. morning erections?
   b. nighttime erections?
   c. erections with masturbation?
   d. erections with partner stimulation (manual)?
   e. erections with partner stimulation (oral)?
      (1) with her mouth on your genitals?
      (2) with your mouth on her genitals?
   f. erections with fantasy only?
   g. erections with intercourse?
   h. erections with extramarital sex?
   i. erections with prostitute experience?
   j. other?

A grade 5 erection is usually sufficient to achieve penetration. Anything less is usually insufficient for insertion. Your scale of erections can tell you many things. If you have good erections in every circumstance except with a woman, the problem is psychological, not physical. If you are erect when doing oral sex to your partner, but not when she is doing it to you, that suggests that you are enjoying yourself when under no pressure to perform. On the other hand, the adrenalin reflex sets in when you feel she is "working" on you.

If you are erect in some situations, but not others, consider your erection as a barometer of your degree of comfort in each circumstance. Think about it and see what conclusions you can draw on your own.

If you are not erect, or only partially erect in all these circumstances, it is highly probable that you are experiencing a physical difficulty and need further medical evaluation.

Widower's syndrome is an exception. It falls into a gray zone. You can have 0 erections in all categories and with appropriate psychotherapy return to good function. A medical evaluation is still required, however.

9: When do you most typically lose erections?

If it is completely unpredictable, you are an exception to the rule. Most men have a pattern that repeats itself; for example, loss at the point of penetration or while changing positions, or during thrusting. If there is a pattern—a certain point when erections are lost—the problem is psychological rather than physical (unless physical pain is responsible—i.e., pain during thrusting).

10: How frequently do you masturbate?

Masturbation does not cause impotence. Some men believe the myth that they are given only so many ejaculations in a lifetime and might use them all up if they have too much sex. This is not true. Most impotent men can masturbate without difficulty. If you masturbate several times a week, you have a better probability of healthy sexual adjustment throughout life than if you do not masturbate at all.

11: Do you fantasize during masturbation? During intercourse?

Men who do not fantasize are more susceptible to having difficulty with erections. If you fantasize with masturbation, but not with intercourse, that may contribute to your inability to be erect with intercourse.

12: What is the state of your general health?

In particular, do you have diabetes, pituitary or thyroid disease, past or present infertility problems, vascular disease, heart disease, neurological disease, or urological disease? Have you had any kidney, bladder, prostate or bowel surgery? These problems and many others can affect your sexuality. However, bear in mind that you can have a disease such as diabetes, and still be impotent for psychological reasons.

13: What medications are you taking?

Many medications influence sex drive and erections. Each medicine needs to be evaluated individually.

14: Do you smoke tobacco? How many packs/day?

We don't know exactly how tobacco affects sex, but we know that nicotine constricts the vessels in your extremities. It can't be good for your erection.

15: Do you drink alcohol? How many ounces/day?

Alcohol slows your sexual reactions. More than two drinks a day can prevent some men from getting erections. If you have any difficulty at all, start treatment at home by eliminating alcohol. If that doesn't work, get professional help.

16: What contraceptive method are you using?

Condoms are the worst for an impotent male and the best for a premature ejaculator. In the time you use fiddling to get it on, the erection can disappear. Once on, the decreased sensation, even if ever so little, doesn't help an impotent man but might delay a premature ejaculator slightly.

17: Grade your relationship or marriage on a 0–10 scale.

If you chose 8 or above, your marriage is not detracting from your sex life. 5–7 is a gray zone. If your marriage scores below 5, and has been there for any length of time, chances are the quality of your relationship is dampening your libido.

18: Do you avoid dating because of sexual difficulties?

If you answered this question affirmatively, you are en route to becoming socially and emotionally isolated. The longer you ignore the problem the more severe it will get.

In your self-assessment of impotence, consider the following: If you have a grade 10 erection under any circumstances, there is no mechanical impairment. If you can masturbate to orgasm with a good erection, *there is nothing physically wrong with you:* it is all in your head. Better to pursue some form of therapy to resolve your problem than to hide from yourself and end up living with it for the rest of your life. A grade 10 erection with masturbation shows no problem. Anything less is questionable.

If you cannot get an erection under any circumstances, it is probably physical. But you cannot know for certain that you get no erections unless you have had the NPT monitoring test done. If you get some degree of erection some of the time, it may be physical or psychological. If you are ejaculating through a flaccid penis some of the time, it could also be either. If you ejaculate through a soft penis all of the time, it is probably physical.

PREMATURE EJACULATION

The following questionnaire is intended to help you determine whether you have the problem of premature ejaculation and whether it is severe enough to require treatment.

1. How long do you last—from the moment of penetration to the moment of ejaculation (in seconds, thrusts, or minutes)?
2. Do you ever ejaculate prior to penetration without meaning to?

3. Have you ever ejaculated without direct physical stimulation of the penis:
   a. under emotional stress, such as during an examination?
   b. under physical stress, like rope climbing?
   c. while fully clothed, from kissing or petting.
4. Do you try to think nonsexual thoughts to distract yourself so that you are able to last longer?
5. Do you skip foreplay hoping to last longer during intercourse?
6. Have you ever tried numbing ointments or other home remedies for premature ejaculation?
7. Do you ejaculate twice (start intercourse again immediately after your first orgasm) hoping to last longer the second time?
8. How long do you think your partner wants you to last?
9. Do you ejaculate more quickly when you are on top than when you are on the bottom?
10. Have you always ejaculated rapidly? If not, when did it begin?
11. Are there some circumstances under which you can last longer:
    a. if you drink alcohol, smoke marijuana, or consume other drugs?
    b. with some women and not others?
12. Do you sometimes lose erections or have difficulty obtaining one?
13. Is your partner hostile and angry with you for ejaculating too soon?

Interpretation

1: How long do you last—from the moment of penetration to the moment of ejaculation (in seconds, thrusts, or minutes)?

If you come in a minute or two, that is probably too brief a time for most women. If you last over ten minutes, you are bordering on lasting too long for most women.

There are many exceptions to both these rules, and it's important to bear in mind that if a woman can't have an orgasm with ten minutes of thrusting, the odds are against her being orgasmic with an hour of thrusting. The duration of your erection is not the problem. There is something else missing.

2: Do you ever ejaculate prior to penetration without meaning to?

Occasionally this happens to every man. He gets so involved in another sexual activity that feels so good, he ejaculates without really meaning to. However, if this occurs more than on a rare occasion, you may be subject to premature ejaculation.

3: Have you ever ejaculated without direct physical stimulation of the penis:

a. under emotional stress, such as during an examination?

b. under physical stress, like rope climbing?

c. while fully clothed, from kissing or petting?

If the answer is yes to one or more of these, the premature ejaculation you are experiencing with intercourse is probably severe enough to require therapy. "Mind over matter" will not be enough.

4: Do you try to think nonsexual thoughts to distract yourself so that you are able to last longer?

This is the most commonly attempted home remedy of all. It generally does not delay ejaculation. However, it will take away the pleasure of the experience. Once you get very, very good at thinking of graveyards, counting backward from a hundred, pinching yourself, biting your cheek—whatever methods you use to tune out your feelings—you will probably succeed in making yourself impotent. Since you are going to ejaculate rapidly anyway, pay attention and enjoy it, until you get some therapy to help you change this pattern.

5: Do you skip foreplay hoping to last longer during intercourse?

Women, given the choice, would rather have the foreplay, the leisure, touching, and intimacy. Chances are, so would you if you will only slow down enough to allow yourself to enjoy it. It does not delay ejaculation to skip foreplay. If you rush through foreplay to prevent premature ejaculation, you are obviously concerned and should get some help.

6: Have you ever tried numbing ointments or other home remedies for premature ejaculation?

This indicates that—whether or not you are a premature ejaculator—you think you are, or are afraid that you are. You may or may not need therapy, but it is wise to consult with an expert and discuss your concerns. If the primary problem is that you think you have a problem, a session or two is often enough to eliminate even a long-standing concern.

7: Do you ejaculate twice (start intercourse again immediately after your first orgasm) hoping to last longer the second time?

If you do, you have probably told yourself that you don't really have a problem because it all works out the second time around. Age will catch up with you. This approach is a short-term solution that is far better than tuning yourself out. However, it does enable you to ignore the problem far longer than you otherwise would. Some women complain that once a man has ejaculated inside of them, thrusting is painful. In some individuals, the mix of secretions causes burning, and intercourse a second time is uncomfortable.

8: How long do you think your partner wants you to last?

Pick a figure out of your imagination; then take the risk and ask her. Don't assume that every woman would want you to last as long as you could. Find out how your partner feels about it and don't discredit that preference by saying, "She doesn't know what she's talking about," or "She is just saying that to be kind."

9: Do you ejaculate more quickly when you are on top than when you are on the bottom?

If so, you are like most men. If you ejaculate equally quickly in both positions, your premature ejaculation may be more severe than most.

10: Have you always ejaculated rapidly? If not, when did it begin?

The vast majority of premature ejaculators have been that way since their first sexual experience. Nothing they have tried to do has helped, except perhaps temporarily. In those men who have developed premature ejaculation later in life—whether gradually or suddenly—the trouble is often associated with the onset of impotence, medical problems such as pain with ejaculation, or perhaps other unusual circumstances.

There is one exception. Men married to aversive women may become premature ejaculators. They are conditioned to ejaculate quickly by wives who say, verbally or nonverbally, "Hurry up and get this over with." Men in this situation often feel they are imposing sexually on the woman and so will hurry as much as they can. After many years of rapid ejaculation, it becomes a conditioned reflex and the man loses the ability to slow down.

11: Are there some circumstances under which you can last longer:

> **a. if you drink alcohol, smoke marijuana, or consume other drugs?**
>
> **b. with some women and not others?**

If a few cocktails or some marijuana slows your speed of ejaculation, the odds are that your rapid ejaculation is primarily related to anxiety. In this case, the adrenalin reflex is exerting its greatest power over you. You are probably a man who is anxious, tense, nervous in general, and tends to perspire a lot with little provocation. Under these circumstances, some stress reduction is needed and—if the premature ejaculation is not too severe—traditional psychotherapy for anxiety can be very effective.

12: Do you sometimes lose erections or have difficulty obtaining one?

If you consider yourself a premature ejaculator and these symptoms are developing, you have waited far too long to get help. Face the problems that rapid ejaculation is causing in your life, and do something about it before you become completely impotent.

13: Is your partner hostile and angry with you for ejaculating too soon?

Women tend to be more understanding of impotence than of premature ejaculation because they don't understand premature ejaculation at all. As a matter of fact, they don't understand impotence very well either.

They feel sympathy for a man who is unable to get erect and sometimes fear that it is their fault. This sympathy-guilt combination prevents them from being too critical.

The man who ejaculates too quickly, however, does not arouse their sympathy. Women are not terribly considerate of premature ejaculators. They erroneously assume that the man is being selfish and thoughtless. He usually cries out in some distress, "I'm coming," when he realizes that he is about to have an orgasm. She thinks: "Well, if you know you're coming, for heaven's sake, why don't you stop." As a woman, she can interrupt her own orgasms, and she is usually not aware of that state of ejaculatory inevitability which, once reached, leaves the man without options. She assumes that he has more control than he is exercising and becomes angry and resentful about it. This, in turn, adds to the man's distress, and he is inclined to ejaculate even more quickly.

Self-Evaluation Questionnaires for Women

Women's sexual difficulties fall into three categories: first, you must find out if there is an actual problem. For example, some women don't know whether or not they are having an orgasm. Determining the nature of their responsiveness is the challenge and, sometimes, the solution.

The second category involves problems arising from expectations—their own and those of the men they are with. A woman may be functioning normally sexually, but her partner isn't pleased. He considers her not responsive enough, and either blames himself and his technique or accuses her of being frigid. Even without an actual problem on her part, stress between them can destroy the entire sexual relationship.

The third category consists of the actual problems, such as difficulty with orgasm or pain with intercourse.

The first questionnaire is the nine-question female screening test. If you answer yes to any of the questions, you should evaluate your situation more carefully by going on to answer the other questionnaires.

The second questionnaire evaluates your expectations and those of your partner; and the final two investigate the differences between psychological sexual difficulties and physical sexual difficulties, and help you determine the specific nature of the problem.

SEXUAL SELF-ASSESSMENT

1. Do you have difficulty having orgasms?
2. Do you think you take too long to have an orgasm?
3. Do you ever find you are working at being orgasmic?
4. Do you have orgasms less than half the time you desire one?
5. Do you have difficulty lubricating?
6. Do you have difficulty becoming aroused?
7. As a rule, do you desire sex more often or less often than your partner?
8. Do you have pain with intercourse?
9. Does your partner have a sexual problem? Does he:
   a. last too long?
   b. ejaculate too quickly?
   c. have difficulty getting or losing erections?

If you have answered yes to *any* of the above questions, you *may* be developing or already have a sexual problem, and should read the interpretation that follows.

Interpretation

1: Do you have difficulty having orgasms?

A positive answer to this question implies that, for whatever reason, you are working at sex. That may be because you have a sexual problem and are trying to correct it. If you have to try to have an orgasm and generally do not succeed, you are not allowing your sexual response to occur as it might naturally. The effort you are making will itself cause a problem, whether there is one to begin with or not.

2: Do you think you take too long to have an orgasm?

If a woman thinks she is taking too long to reach a climax, she is usually worried about her partner becoming bored or tired (she already is). This concern alone will cause her to take still longer. If she generally takes more than half an hour to become orgasmic, that is longer than is biologically necessary. Most women who are fully functional can have an orgasm within fifteen minutes or less. However, remember that this is not a race—there are no world records to be met. Women who can be orgasmic in nanoseconds may prefer on occasion to take hours.

Think of how long it takes you to get to orgasm when you masturbate. Sex with a partner shouldn't take you significantly longer.

3: Do you ever find you are working at being orgasmic?

If, during sex, the thought crosses your mind that "I wish he would get it over with," or "This is too much work," or "It is taking too long," or "No matter how hard I try, or what I do, it won't work," you are working too hard. You cannot expect to respond under those circumstances.

4: Do you have orgasms less than half the time you desire one?

Once a woman knows what an orgasm feels like, she should be able to have one rather easily. Most men and women have little difficulty masturbating once they learn how. Ninety percent of the time they can count on reaching orgasm eventually—unless there is either a sexual problem or an unusual circumstance of some sort. Therefore, once you are functioning well sexually with your partner, you should be able to count on a normal response much of the time.

5: Do you have difficulty lubricating?

Women who have difficulty becoming lubricated are either not aroused or there is something physically wrong with them. Physical problems which limit lubrication are exceedingly rare prior to menopause, unless there is also pain associated with intercourse. Women in pain rarely lubricate.

6: Do you have difficulty becoming aroused?

There are several possible causes to this problem: you may be aversive, you may be trying too hard, or you may be so angry or disappointed with your partner that sex is not very appealing. Another possibility is that you are so unaware of your sexual and sensual self that you are ignorant of how to become involved.

7: As a rule, do you desire sex more often or less often than your partner?

If your partner consistently wants sex more or less often than you do, the stress and pressure associated with the initiation of sex can be sufficient to cause two people to avoid sex altogether. Sexual aversion is the eventual outcome.

8: Do you have pain with intercourse?

Pain of any sort that lasts for any period of time can prevent you from becoming aroused. It is possible to enjoy sex in spite of the pain, but the more severe the distress, the less chance there is of that happening. In short, don't expect to enjoy it if it hurts.

Women who find pelvic examinations painful usually also have pain with intercourse. A pelvic examination should not hurt unless there is something wrong with you (or your doctor).

9: Does your partner have a sexual problem? Does he:
a. last too long?
b. ejaculate too quickly?
c. have difficulty getting or losing erections?

If your partner is a premature ejaculator or is impotent, although it is *his* dysfunction it is *your* distress. It can cause you to have problems in your sexual response. Or, if you already had difficulty in having an orgasm, his problems will allow you to hide from your own. It is, after all, technically "his fault." When you hide behind his dysfunction, you may not address your own.

EXPECTATIONS

1. How would you like to respond sexually? How do you think your partner would like you to respond?

2. Describe your impression of your ideal sexual response.

3. How often would you like to be having intercourse?
a. How often are you actually having intercourse?
b. How often do you think your partner would like to have intercourse?

4. How long would you like your partner to thrust before ejaculating?
a. Approximately how long does he last?
b. How long do you think he would like to last?

5. What percentage of the time would you like to be orgasmic?
a. What percentage of the time are you orgasmic?
b. What percentage of the time do you think your partner would like you to be orgasmic?

Interpretation

1: How would you like to respond sexually? How do you think your partner would like you to respond?

After you have answered both parts of the question compare your answers. Are your goals similar or different from your impression of your partner's? Ask your partner to describe changes he would like and see how they compare to your perception of his preferences. Review the changes you have described. Are they realistic? Reread the sections in Chapter 1, where unrealistic sexual expectations are described in some detail, and make sure that you have come to terms with reality.

2: Describe your impression of your ideal sexual response.

If your description reveals the best of our most torrid popular novelists, chances are you are putting unrealistic pressure on your sexual aspirations. On the other hand, if, in addition to the specifics, you place a high priority on comfort, fun, leisure, communication, and intimacy, your expectations exist in a favorable setting.

3: How often would you like to be having intercourse?
 a. How often are you actually having intercourse?
 b. How often do you think your partner would like to have intercourse?

Frequency of intercourse commonly ranges from once a week to once a day. Few couples sustain the pace of once a day indefinitely, but some do. Sex will not be frequent in a hostile environment. If you are overextended, fatigued, and are making no effort to change the pressures in your life, improving the quality and frequency of your sex life is unrealistic. If you change the setting by reevaluating your priorities, increasing your sexual frequency becomes a realistic possibility.

4: How long would you like your partner to thrust before ejaculating?
 a. Approximately how long does he last?
 b. How long do you think he would like to last?

The length of time men last varies from seconds to hours. The common range is a few minutes to half an hour. Longer is not necessarily better, especially if sex has become a project—"Operation Orgasm." If that half-hour is a means to an end rather than an end in itself the quality of your sex life is suffering.

5: What percentage of the time would you like to be orgasmic?

    a. What percentage of the time are you orgasmic?

    b. What percentage of the time do you think your partner would like you to be orgasmic?

If you are hoping for 100 percent you are probably going to be disappointed. The survey studies show that only 40 percent of women are orgasmic with intercourse at all although they may be orgasmic in other ways. If you are preoccupied with being orgasmic with every sexual experience, much less hoping to have mutual orgasms consistently, your goals are basically unrealistic. However, frequent orgasms, multiple orgasms, and mutual orgasms can occur often if you are living up to and fulfilling your sexual potential.

IS IT PHYSICAL OR PSYCHOLOGICAL?

The Psychological Screen

If you have had orgasms, but not with partner manipulation and/or intercourse, ask yourself the following questions:

1. Have you ever experienced orgasm by any means?
    a. dream state?
    b. masturbation?
    c. partner stimulation?
    d. intercourse?
    e. vibrator?
    f. other?
2. What method do you use for masturbation? (Manual, object, etc.)
    a. How long does it take you to be orgasmic with masturbation?
    b. Have you experienced more than one orgasm at a time by any method?
3. Does your partner do anything that causes you physical discomfort? Do you tell him about it or do you endure it?
4. Do you ever fake orgasm or exaggerate your sexual response?
5. What are you thinking about during sex?

6. Are you easily distracted during sex?
7. How often did you have sex this past year?
    a. Is it more or less than in previous years?
    b. Would you like it to be more or less than it is?
8. Do you enjoy having sex?
9. Do you feel under pressure to have more sex?

Interpretation

1: Have you ever experienced orgasm by any means?

If you have been orgasmic by *any* method, you are wired together correctly. Your systems are intact.

2: What method do you use for masturbation? (Manual, object, etc.)

    a. How long does it take you to be orgasmic with masturbation?

However long it takes you with masturbation is how short it can take you with a partner, if you stop editing.

    b. Have you experienced more than one orgasm at a time by any method?

If you have been multiorgasmic under any circumstances, you are biologically capable and you should be able to learn how to translate that ability to whatever method you choose.

3: Does your partner do anything that causes you physical discomfort? Do you tell him about it or do you endure it?

If your partner's touch is too heavy in the wrong place, don't count on enjoying fantastic sex. The sad fact is that hordes of women endure uncomfortable forms of stimulation while asking themselves innocently, "Why can't I respond?" If there is any physical pain present, there may be something physically wrong with you. In either instance, where there is physical pain, there is a physical problem. You can't expect to enjoy sex when it hurts.

4: Do you ever fake orgasm or exaggerate your sexual response?

If you do, you are probably under some degree of pressure to perform—and if you can't perform naturally, you may fake the response you feel you ought to have. This performance pressure alone is enough to inhibit you psychologically from responding naturally.

5: What are you thinking about during sex?

If you are not having sexual thoughts, you probably won't have sexual reactions.

6: Are you easily distracted during sex?

Women are normally more easily distracted during sex than are men. If you keep thinking, "Oh, the bedroom door is unlocked," "The phone is not off the hook," or "The children may wander in at any moment," it's little wonder you can't concentrate on enjoying the sex.

7: How often did you have sex this past year?
    a. Is it more or less than in previous years?
    b. Would you like it to be more or less than it is?

If your sexual frequency has dropped by a third or more from its high point, be suspicious of sexual aversion.

8: Do you enjoy having sex?

If you are not enjoying sex, and there is no physical problem, there are problems brewing. They are psychological in nature and may involve aspects of your relationship beyond sex.

9: Do you feel under pressure to have more sex?

If you feel under pressure to have sex, aversion is already well advanced. The longer you wait, the worse it will get.

IS IT PHYSICAL OR PSYCHOLOGICAL?

The Physiological Screen

If you are not orgasmic by any method, or if it feels different or takes you much longer than it used to, ask yourself the following questions:

1. What is your general state of health?
2. What medical illnesses have you had?
3. Have you ever had surgery on your genitals, pelvis, or abdominal organs?
   a. Were there any complications?
   b. Were any of them related to the problems you have developed?
4. Does it take longer to be orgasmic than it used to?
5. Are your orgasms less intense and/or less frequent today than they used to be?

6. Has the duration of your orgasms changed recently?
7. Were these changes gradual or sudden?
8. Were these changes related to:
   a. marriage?
   b. pregnancy?
   c. birth of a child?
   d. an extramarital affair?
9. Do you ever have physical pain during sexual activity?
   a. Do you ever have any discomfort of any kind with sexual activity?
   b. How often?
10. When did you experience menopause? Was it surgical or natural?
11. What drugs are you taking? What medicines are you taking? How much alcohol do you drink each day?

Interpretation

1: What is your general state of health?

If you are fatigued, tired, depressed, dizzy, headachy, premenstrual, etc., your sexual life will be negatively affected.

2: What medical illnesses have you had?

Some problems directly affect sex, such as diabetes and multiple sclerosis. Other medical problems affect sex indirectly by making you feel generally unwell—arthritis, emphysema, hepatitis.

3: Have you ever had surgery on your genitals, pelvis, or abdominal organs?

    a. Were there any complications?

    b. Were any of them related to problems you have developed?

Hysterectomies, bowel surgeries, and sometimes even exploratory surgeries can sever nerves that will disrupt your sexual functioning.

4: Does it take longer to be orgasmic than it used to?

If it does, this suggests one of two things. Either your attitude and relationship are changing for the worse, or some physical problem could be developing.

5: Are your orgasms less intense and/or less frequent today than they used to be?

Other than menopause—which will normally diminish the

degree of orgasmic intensity in small increments—diminution of intensity can mean a possible physical problem. It can be psychological, too. If you don't pay attention, intensity diminishes. If frequency decreases, it is usually psychological, unless pain or discomfort is responsible.

6: Has the duration of your orgasms changed recently?

Again, with the exception of menopause, if your orgasms are shorter in duration than they need to be, physical changes may be occurring.

7: Were these changes gradual or sudden?

A sudden change in the ability to respond is suggestive of a psychological cause. Gradual and insidious changes can also be psychological, but are usually characteristic of physical problems.

8: Were these changes related to:
   a. marriage?
   b. pregnancy?
   c. birth of child?
   d. extramarital affair?

Changes related to marriage and extramarital affairs are generally psychological in nature. Changes related to pregnancy and/or delivery of the child can be either physical or psychological. A pregnancy can be accompanied by physical complications (often arising during delivery) that can have residual effects. The doctor who delivers your baby may, without your knowledge, take a "love stitch" that makes you so tight that sex becomes painful. More frequently, pregnancy and delivery precipitate psychological problems that interfere with a good sexual relationship.

9: Do you ever have physical pain during sexual activity?
   a. Do you ever have any discomfort of any kind with sexual activity?
   b. How often?

Many women who say no to the pain question will admit they occasionally have discomfort that they disregard. They assume it is probably lack of lubrication or some other temporary malfunction. On closer questioning, they realize that the discomfort is there most of the time, and that it successfully interferes with their sexual response.

10: When did you experience menopause? Was it surgical or natural?

Menopause has unpredictable effects on a woman's sexual responsiveness but needs to be considered as a landmark—a period from which precise symptoms can be studied. Look at the years during which you progressed through menopause and ask yourself what sexual changes occurred and whether they were related to your present problem.

11: What drugs are you taking? What medicines are you taking? How much alcohol do you drink each day?

The effects of drugs, medications, and alcohol on a woman's sexual libido and responsiveness are far less clearly defined than for the man. Until science can provide more distinct guidelines, you must assess each of these factors on an individual basis. If you find that alcohol suppresses your libido, don't drink. If you find that Valium depresses everything, stop taking it. In the area of medication, birth control pills, and female hormones, you are on your own. You must be a conscientious consumer. Exercise good judgment and be cautious.

From Expectations to Realizations

If you ask yourself the right questions, you can't help but come up with some of the right answers. It is when you too readily allow other people to answer your questions that you get misled. We'll consider several levels in which problems can occur.

In an attempt to understand your problems, you must first determine if the problem is a figment of your imagination (or his). At that level, the problem can be just as real as a specific dysfunction—but it is different. If you are a sexually well-adjusted female and have no trouble reaching orgasms, that's fine. But, if he expects you to tap-dance about with a rose between your teeth during sex there could be a problem. His expectations become your frustrations.

If you, the man, enjoy sex, take a leisurely pace, savor touching, and last—in your opinion—a reasonable length of time, also fine. Now, suppose she demands that you thrust for hours and preferably several times a day. Then it is her expectation that's creating your problem.

If your sex life is good, you'll have to work hard (and enjoyably) to keep it that way. If it isn't good, the sooner you correct the problem the less damage it can do to your otherwise good relationship. If both your sex life and your relationship are in serious trouble, that does not mean automatically that you need to trade partners, that the relationship is bad. It may mean that both of you are ill-equipped to function successfully and maturely in *any* relationship—shown by the fact that you have gotten into so much trouble in this one.

If you muster your resources and make an effort, you will be surprised at how dramatically you can improve an apparently "hopeless" situation.

ABOUT THE AUTHOR

Theresa Larsen Crenshaw, M.D., is one of a handful of dedicated women physicians specializing in sexual medicine. Dr. Crenshaw is co-director of the Division of Human Sexuality, Department of Reproductive Medicine (Obstetrics and Gynecology), University of California, San Diego School of Medicine, and also Vice-President of the American Association of Sex Educators, Counselors and Therapists. Dr. Crenshaw is a graduate of Stanford University and the University of California, Irvine, Medical School. She received her specialty training from Dr. William Masters and Virginia Johnson, and is currently the Director of The Crenshaw Clinic in San Diego, which she founded.

Dr. Crenshaw has published dozens of scientific papers, currently writes a newspaper column of advice on sexual problems, lectures nationally, and is widely sought after by the media.